Overcome the Challenges
of Cancer Care

Overcome the Challenges of Cancer Care

How to Avoid Pitfalls on the Path to Healing

Stephen Rosenberg, MD

ROWMAN & LITTLEFIELD
Lanham • Boulder • New York • London

Published by Rowman & Littlefield
An imprint of The Rowman & Littlefield Publishing Group, Inc.
4501 Forbes Boulevard, Suite 200, Lanham, Maryland 20706
www.rowman.com

6 Tinworth Street, London SE11 5AL, United Kingdom

British Library Cataloguing in Publication Information Available

Library of Congress Cataloging-in-Publication Data

Names: Stephen Rosenberg
Title: Overcome the challenges of cancer care : How to avoid pitfalls on the path to healing
Description: Lanham : Rowman & Littlefield [2020] / Includes bibliographical references and index. / Summary: "A friendly, easy-to-read guide for cancer patients and their loved ones when dealing with a cancer diagnosis. This book will help patients, loved ones, friends and family recognize the pitfalls of a cancer diagnosis and how to avoid them to get the best care possible during their cancer journey." --Provided by publisher.
Identifiers: LCCN 2019051825 (print) / LCCN 2019051826 (ebook) / ISBN 9781538134221 (cloth) / ISBN 9781538134238 (epub)
Subjects: LCSH: Cancer--Patients--Care. / Cancer--Patients--Rehabilitation. / Cancer--Treatment.
Classification: LCC RC262.R655 2020 (print) / LCC RC262 (ebook) / DDC 616.99/4--dc23
LC record available at https://lccn.loc.gov/2019051825
LC ebook record available at https://lccn.loc.gov/2019051826

For my wife, Katie
son, Jonathan
daughter, Emily
parents, Allen and Dorothy
and everyone touched by cancer

Contents

Preface

Early in my medical training, I tried to direct patients to resources about cancer. The books patients found were, overwhelming, poorly written or just plain false. As patients went online, they found a mix of half-truths and false promises.

I did my best to educate my patients in clinic. But even with an hour-long patient visit, I didn't feel like I could convey everything I needed to. I wrote this book because I was distraught by the lack of quality information available to patients. The goal of this book is to fill in the *who*, *what*, *when*, *where*, and *why* of cancer in an easy-to-read format.

We've all been touched by cancer—a spouse, a brother, a mother, a sister, a friend, or even ourselves. Each year in the United States, there are about 1.7 million new cancer cases and about 600,000 deaths from cancer. It is the second most common cause of death in the United States, behind only heart disease. Cancer plays some role in almost everyone's life, so I hope to shed light on this common but devastating disease.

Some books examine every nuance of cancer for hundreds of pages. Wading through the sea of information can bring shock and panic to patients and loved ones. That's why this book is not comprehensive. I only briefly touch on individual cancers. Instead, I focus on the processes and treatment of cancer as a whole. I want to make sure you or your loved ones don't miss the forest for the trees.

I hope you find this book useful and informative. I would love to hear your thoughts on the book.

Warm regards,
Stephen Rosenberg, MD
stephen.rosenberg.md@gmail.com

Introduction

"You have cancer."

When people hear these words, they're at a loss. *How could this happen? What do I do now? Where do I begin?* These are only some of the questions patients, family members, and others have.

The average person has a limited view of what cancer is, how it grows, and how we treat it. People hear things about cancer on TV, read about it in books, and see people deal with it in movies. Many of us even donate time and money to cancer research. But we often talk about cancer in a superficial sense. We rarely dive into what it means to have cancer or how to deal with it.

Maybe we hear about a friend or family member who has cancer: "Uncle Bob has prostate cancer" or "Aunt Susan has breast cancer." We think, *That's too bad.* Maybe, in the quiet and privacy of our homes, we Google the word *cancer*. The amount of information overloads us. (By the way, if you do Google the word *cancer*, you get over half a billion results.)

Taking in a diagnosis while wading through this information is overwhelming.

WHERE DO I START?

As you work through information online and in books from doctors, healers, salespeople, and anyone in between, the picture only gets cloudier. Worse yet, there are a lot of false promises and poorly written materials out there. Some people try to exploit patients, families, and friends affected by cancer.

I hope this book serves as a guide—a flashlight in the darkness of cancer information. I want to arm you with information on cancer in an easy-to-understand format.

We'll start with the cancer cell, describe diagnosis, and go over the types of common treatments: surgery, chemotherapy, radiation, and immunotherapy. We'll then move on to managing side effects, incorporating complementary care, and making lifestyle changes. Throughout the book, I also outline how to overcome the ten most common mistakes I see patients and families make as they go through this process.

At the end, I've included a glossary, where you can find definitions of terms, and a list of additional resources. Please also visit my website at stephenrosenbergmd.com where I've included patient resources, such as templates for doctor's appointments with questions to ask along with other helpful lists. I want you to have everything you or family members may need to navigate the journey of cancer.

GETTING THE BIG PICTURE

This book isn't a comprehensive course on cancer, as there are many types of cancer. In fact, you can find entire textbooks devoted to breast cancer, prostate cancer, or many other types of cancer!

Many of these books drag patients down into the details of cancer without giving them the big picture—the "Where is this going?" My goal is to provide an overview of cancer. I want you to understand how cancer grows, how we treat it, and how to move forward.

With that in mind, let's get started.

Chapter One

Cancer 101

This chapter provides a broad overview of what cancer is, including where it comes from and how to think about it. Cancer is just a shadow of us. To get to know cancer, we need to get to know ourselves.

CANCER: MILLIONS OF DISEASES

Cancer is *not* one disease. It's millions of them. It varies from person to person and even *within* the same person. We see a huge range in *prognosis* (the course a disease will take) and patients' survival times.

Suppose a woman named Leslie develops a breast cancer, and so does her neighbor Jill. The biology (behavior) of Leslie's cancer is going to be different from Jill's. Leslie's cancer may respond to chemotherapy, while Jill's cancer may not. Such differences make it hard to come up with a single cure for cancer.

Overall, cancer death rates have declined, and the number of cancer survivors has increased. This is great news! But it does mean we need to look at the long-term effects of cancer and its treatment.

WHERE IN THE BODY DOES CANCER COME FROM?

Cancer comes from almost anywhere in the body. No organ or cell is immune from turning into cancer.

Cancer, at its core, comes from cells, which are the building blocks of your body. The average human body is made up of 30 to 40 trillion cells. Each cell has a *nucleus*, which you can think of as the control center or brain of the cell.

Stored in the nucleus is the *DNA*. DNA contains the genes that make up who and what you are. These genes are the instruction manuals for a cell. Cancer comes from mistakes made in copying the DNA. (See the glossary for a scientific definition of *DNA*.)

MUTATIONS ARE THE DRIVERS OF CANCER

Mutations are changes to DNA, the brain of the cell. These changes underlie the process a normal cell undergoes when it becomes a cancer cell. Mutations in DNA lead to abnormal instructions being sent to the rest of the cell.

Some risk factors for mutations include age, smoking, alcohol, weight gain, certain infections (such as HPV and hepatitis B or C), environmental exposures, genetics, and lots of other factors we don't yet understand. Many of these risk factors mess with our DNA in inappropriate ways that lead to cancer.

Environmental causes of cancer include exposure to certain chemicals and other materials (these are called *carcinogens*—see the glossary for a scientific definition). An example of an environmental factor that can cause cancer is asbestos. Exposure to asbestos puts people at risk for a type of lung cancer (*mesothelioma*).

WHY AGE IS A RISK FOR CANCER

Age is one of the biggest risk factors for cancer. We see cancer much more commonly in older people compared to young people.

Each time a cell divides, it has to make a copy of its DNA. Random errors occur in the DNA during the copying process. This is a normal part of existence. Most of the time, the cell corrects these errors. As a cell gets older, it makes errors more often and corrects them less often. Therefore, the chance of mutation (changes in DNA) increases over time!

CANCER CELLS GROW LIKE WEEDS:
UNLIMITED GROWTH IN THE GARDEN

Errors in DNA can cause cells to behave selfishly. The faulty DNA tells the rest of the cancer cell to divide (split into two cells). In simple terms, one cell becomes two, two cells become four, four cells become eight, and so on. After ten divisions, that one cell has led to more than a thousand others! This is where we get the definition for *cancer*—a disease caused by the unchecked growth (or division) of cells in the body.

Like weeds in a garden, cancer cells take up valuable space and resources in organs. Cancer cells push on the normal cells, leading to abnormal function of the normal cells of that organ. This may lead to terrible consequences for patients.

SOLID TUMORS

In general, we split cancers into two types: *liquid tumors* and *solid tumors*. Knowing which type of tumor we're dealing with gives us information on how a cancer may behave.

Solid tumors are cancers that originate in any solid organ or structure in the body. This could be the lung, the liver, or even the heart! Solid tumors can (and unfortunately do) spread to other parts of the body. The movement of cancer cells from one part of the body to another is called *metastasis*.

With a solid tumor, cancer cells originate from a mass or lesion (compared to liquid tumors, which come from the bone marrow; see the next section). This mass may be cut out with surgery or treated with radiation, chemotherapy, or some combination of the two.

LIQUID TUMORS

Liquid tumors are cancers that make their home in the bloodstream. These cancers include the many types of leukemia.

The cells in your blood (liquid) come from the *bone marrow*. The bone marrow makes up the inside of large bones, such as the pelvis or spine.

The normal cells made in the bone marrow are vital for normal function of the human body. These cells include *red blood cells*, which carry oxygen throughout the body; *white blood cells*, which are the immune cells that fight infections; and *platelets*, which are cells that allow the blood to clot.

Mutations in the cells of the bone marrow often lead to these liquid tumors. Because blood moves throughout your body, these cells may travel anywhere blood goes. This makes surgery, which focuses on only one part of the body, less likely to be part of the treatment.

These definitions of solid and liquid tumors are useful, but they aren't perfect. For example, a cancer called *lymphoma* falls in between: it forms masses in the lymph nodes but is often thought of as a liquid tumor. We'll talk about lymph nodes later on.

HOW DOES CANCER DECIDE WHERE TO GO?

Cancer spreads anywhere it needs to go to find an environment with resources to help it grow. It's clear that different types of cancers tend to spread to certain parts of the body. For example, prostate cancer tends to spread to bone. Breast cancer tends to spread to the armpit region (lymph nodes are hidden there). Lung cancers often spread in the chest or to the brain.

These patterns of spread can be very specific. Just like there are certain soils that are better for some plants, there are better places in the body for certain cancers to grow. This idea is called the *seed and soil hypothesis*. These specific patterns happen because cancer cells communicate with (send signals to) other organs.

WHERE HAS ALL THE PROGRESS GONE?

We've been waging the "war on cancer" since 1971 (it started with the Nixon administration). Patients often express frustration at the lack of progress in treating cancer. Where has all that money in cancer research gone? Why aren't we doing better?

First, let me say that doctors are frustrated too. We've definitely made strides in treating cancer, but we have a long way to go.

Treating cancer is hard for many reasons. One is that when cancer spreads to different parts of the body, it can keep on changing. As cancer cells grow, new changes in the DNA may allow them to grow faster.

Cancer is like a weed. A weed will use any advantage to go after sunlight, water, and nutrients in the soil. In the same way, a cancer cell will use any competitive edge for resources in the body. Weeds do this by growing taller and faster than many other plants to gain more access to sunlight. The deep roots of weeds are difficult to remove, allowing the weed to regrow if it breaks. Cancer cells, like weeds, will try to steal the nutrients from normal organs and cells need to survive. The changes cancer cells go through also allow them to be more resistant to chemotherapy, radiation, or immunotherapy.

Another problem is that cancer cells are so much like normal cells; they're like closely related cousins. Most of the DNA between a normal cell and a cancer cell is the same. It can be hard to tell the cells apart.

In a garden, you want to make sure any method you use to get rid of weeds—pulling them out, spraying weed killer, etc.—doesn't remove the local plants too. But at its core, a weed is still a plant. To get rid of weeds, you need to figure out what makes weeds different from other plants. In the same way, the only way to treat cancer is to find some differences between normal cells and cancer cells. Finding and exploiting these differences for treatments is hard.

CANCER'S ACHILLES' HEEL

Cancer cells have a deep desire to grow and divide. It drives everything they do.

This constant drive to divide is something we use to our benefit in trying to eradicate it. It's the difference between cancer cells and normal cells. Taking advantage of the cancer's basic instincts to divide is why chemotherapy and radiation are effective treatments. Some mutations (changes) in the DNA that allow cancer cells to grow also give us unique targets to hit with our expanding list of drugs. We'll explore this idea in later chapters on types of cancer treatments.

GETTING BACK TO THE BASICS

To summarize, cancer is common. It's the unchecked division of cells in the body caused by mutations. These mutations happen because of age, exposures (known and unknown), and lifestyle choices.

Treating cancer is hard because it's different in different people. It can move to a new part of the body and keep changing. At its core, cancer is just a shadow of us. The cancer cell has a lot in common with a normal cell. But for treatment, we use the cancer's desire to divide against it.

In the next chapter, we'll go back to basic biology to further discuss how cancer grows in relation to normal cells. This will give you some context on how cancer therapies work and what their side effects are.

Chapter Two

The Biology of Cancer

To understand the basics of cancer treatment, you need to understand the biology of cancer. With this goal in mind, we'll review some basic human and cell biology to help you grasp cancer's behavior. Don't worry; we'll keep the science at a sixth- to eighth-grade level. Cancer plays by its own rules, and we'll outline some of these rules as we go.

HOW A NORMAL CELL BEHAVES

Cells are the building blocks of our bodies. Each cell has a nucleus (the center of the cell) that stores the DNA, the "brain" of the cell. The DNA stays in the nucleus, giving out orders.

DNA stores the instruction manual for each one of us. The DNA needs to convey that information to other parts of the cell, so pieces of those instructions are transcribed, or rewritten, as *RNA*. The RNA exits the nucleus, and the RNA's instructions are used to build proteins in the rest of the cell. Proteins then perform the actions of the cell. In short, the information is copied and used in this order:

$$DNA \rightarrow RNA \rightarrow protein$$

The goal of the DNA is to get the instructions to the protein to carry out actions around the cell. These actions could include instructions to grow, divide, sleep, or anything in between.

Each of our normal cells has a program to tell it to stop growing and die when too much damage occurs to the genetic code (the DNA). This process of self-destruction is known as *apoptosis*. Cancer cells lack the normal signals telling them to self-destruct.

The process is much more complicated than this, but this explanation gives you a framework for how cells work. You can find the biological definitions of DNA, RNA, and proteins in the glossary at the back of the book.

MY MOM HAD CANCER . . . WILL I GET CANCER?

Many patients and family members want to know about their genetic risk of getting cancer. If their mom or dad had cancer, will they definitely get cancer?

Most cancers that occur are random events. They come from a mix of risk factors, like age and exposures in the environment such as smoking. (If you're smoking, please stop! See chapter 12, on nutrition and lifestyle, for help.) For many cancers, there is likely some genetic component underlying its development. However, it's only a small part of the risk compared to lifestyle, age, and other factors.

There are genetic syndromes, passed down from parents that increase the risk of getting cancer. These genetic syndromes are *rare*. Still, they do put people at risk for cancer at a much higher rate. Patients may inherit these risks from mom or dad. An example is a mutation in the genes *BRCA1* and *BRCA2* that increases the risk for breast cancer and other cancers.

To avoid cancer, some patients with genetic syndromes decide to have organs taken out before cancer develops. Patients with BRCA1/2 mutations may have both breasts and ovaries removed to significantly reduce that risk. This is because these patients are at very high risk of getting a cancer of these organs.

If you or someone you love has multiple family members with cancer, please discuss this with a doctor. By talking to a doctor, you can help make sure you or a loved one get referred for proper genetic testing. Identifying these genetic syndromes may be important for a cancer patient's siblings or children. A patient should work out a complete family health history before meeting with a cancer doctor.

THE CANCER CELL: MAKING CRAZY DECISIONS

Mutations are what drive cancer. They may come from a random event or damage from the environment. These mutations drive certain behaviors in cancer cells that are unusual.

Imagine that DNA is someone who owns and runs a company. What happens if the owner comes to work not thinking right? Maybe they got bonked on the head and have a concussion or amnesia. In some way, the owner has changed their thinking. Their thinking has *mutated*.

The owner keeps handing down instructions that don't make good sense to the company's managers. Still, the managers pass on those instructions to the employees, who act on them.

This change in thinking corresponds to a mutation in the DNA of a cancer cell. The DNA gives inappropriate instructions to the RNA, which uses them to make the proteins that act throughout the cell.

In the rest of this chapter, I outline the core behaviors of cancer. If you want a technical explanation, check out the paper by Douglas Hanahan and Robert Weinberg listed in the resources at the end of this book.

BUSINESS PARTNERS: KEEPING THE OWNER IN LINE

When cell growth gets out of control, the body has a few systems in place to stop it.

Again, imagine the DNA of a mutated cell as the owner of a company, who's suffering from amnesia after getting hit on the head. So the owner tells the managers to open new stores or to order more inventory, even though the company doesn't have enough money to do that. Luckily, the owner's business partners will try to stop, or suppress, the owner from making these big mistakes. They try to put the brakes on the owner's awful decisions. There are checks and balances in a company to keep it operating smoothly.

There are checks and balances in a cell as well. For example, *tumor suppressors* stop the cell's signal to keep growing. Just like the name implies, they suppress or stop tumors from forming. The most well-known tumor suppressor, p53, is known as the "guardian of the genome."

KICKING OUT THE BUSINESS PARTNERS:
THE CANCER TAKES CHARGE

The business owner in our example doesn't realize anything is wrong! It's annoying having the partners mess with their work. Therefore, the owner gets rid of the partners and runs the company alone.

Now that the partners are gone, there's no one to stop the owner. The owner is clear to keep handing instructions down the chain of command.

In cell terms, the cancer cell gets rid of the tumor suppressors. This may be done through mutations. Once the cancer finds ways around the tumor suppressors, it's free to do what it wants. This allows the cancer cell to focus on growing and dividing.

This is the basic process of cancer growth.

CANCER ORDERS IN: GORGING ON SUGAR

For cancer cells to keep on growing, they need nutrients: sugar and oxygen (just like the rest of us). To help bring in extra supplies, cancer cells demand that the body form new blood vessels directed to the cancer. These vessels bring in sugar and oxygen.

The cancer cell uses sugar in an inefficient way. Because the cancer cell constantly needs energy, it must bring in and use lots of sugar—an endless process. In biology, this idea is called the *Warburg effect* (see glossary).

When looking for cancer cells, we use the Warburg effect to our advantage. A PET scan involves tracking a labeled sugar that is taken up by cancer cells. The labeled sugar shows up on our scans, helping us see where cancer may be located throughout the body.

I discuss PET scans in chapter 3, on diagnosis. Chapter 12 discusses whether cancer patients should avoid sugar in their diet.

NOT KNOWING WHEN TO STOP

Normal cells in your body have self-control. For example, if a normal cell senses damage to its DNA, the cell hits the stop button—it stops growing. This is called *cell cycle arrest*.

A cancer cell is like someone with a drinking problem that keeps getting worse. Each opportunity for the cell to divide is like another drink. These cells don't know when to stop. Even if they're sick or broke, they always ask for one more round. As cancer cells grow, they don't care about damage or other tissues; all they care about is the chance to keep dividing. And just as continuing to drink can further hurt someone's thinking, mutations can lead to more mutations and instability in the cell. More mutations may give cancer cells more advantages to grow over time.

THE UNWELCOME HOUSEGUEST: CANCER MOVES IN

If cancer stayed in one place, it would be way less scary. Unfortunately, cancer finds ways to move from one part of the body to the next. This movement is known as *metastasis*.

When trying to understand metastasis, think of cancer as an unwelcome houseguest. It invades your personal space, taking up precious resources like food without bringing anything positive in return.

The unwelcome guest crashes on the couch, eats all your food, and then asks for more! As cancer spreads to almost any part of the body (say, a bone or organ), it keeps on growing and dividing. There is no signal telling it to stop. Because of this, the cancer may interrupt the normal function of an organ or that part of the body. This is what makes cancer lethal.

Not all cancers are likely to spread. For example, many types of skin cancers rarely metastasize. Tumors that don't spread may meet the definition of cancer (unchecked cell growth) but are much less likely to cause death.

CANCER CELLS DON'T AGE

As we grow older, we get wrinkles and show signs of time's toll on our bodies. But cancer cells don't play by the same rules; they do not age. Cancer cells can invade our organs and use our resources indefinitely.

If we grow cancer cells in a lab dish with appropriate nutrients, they'll grow forever. On the other hand, if we do the same thing with normal cells (even with enough nutrients), they'll eventually stop growing.

How do cancer cells do this?

When cells divide to make new cells, they lose a little bit of DNA each time. This is normal: to ensure you don't lose anything important,

DNA includes some scrap material. Protective ends of your DNA—called *telomeres*—help prevent damage to the necessary parts of the DNA. In normal cells, these protective ends get shorter with age (after each cell division). Just as tree rings give away the age of a tree, the shortening of telomeres gives away the age of a cell. Eventually, a normal cell can't divide anymore as its telomeres get too short to protect DNA, and the cell dies.

Every cell produces a protein known as *telomerase* that repairs the DNA's protective ends. In a cancer cell's mutated DNA, more telomerase is produced than usual. This allows cancer cells to indefinitely protect their DNA ends and avoid the aging process.

IMMUNE-SYSTEM EVASION: HIDING IN PLAIN SIGHT

Part of the immune system's job is to look for any new cancers or precancerous cells and destroy them. This is happening all the time in our bodies.

In the human body, the immune system acts like the police. In fact, the immune system is always on patrol looking for cancer. But cancer cells have ways to keep the immune system from recognizing them. By avoiding the immune system, the cancer can keep on growing.

Cancer cells avoid the immune system by throwing up smoke screens. These cells can also get part of the immune system to help the cancer grow!

How does it do this? The cancer tricks another type of immune cell into destroying the immune cell that was going to destroy the cancer. This is kind of like when internal affairs arrests a good cop, preventing the cop from arresting the criminal (cancer).

BIOLOGY: THE BIG PICTURE

To summarize, cancer cells are just reflections of our normal cells. Information in cancer cells is moved from the nucleus (DNA) to other parts of the cell. Abnormal cell "thinking" leads to strange instructions being sent throughout the cell. A cancer cell's only concern is getting enough oxygen and sugar to go on to its next cell division. Cancer cells may move into other areas of the body and take over—or metastasize—to get the necessary nutrients. Cancer can evade the immune system and overcome the aging process.

Now that you understand how cancer cells behave, we can use that information to help identify cancer. We'll dive into the diagnosis of cancer in the next chapter.

Chapter Three

How Cancer Is Diagnosed

Cancer is sneaky, which can make diagnosing cancer a real challenge. Many of the symptoms of cancers are nonspecific, which means the symptoms could point to a lot of different diseases. Often, it's hard to know whether cancer is the cause of any particular symptom. This can lead to significant delays in the diagnosis of cancer. These delays often make patients feel frustrated and angry.

Cancer cells are so closely related to normal cells that it can be hard to find the differences. To understand each patient's cancer, doctors use information from biopsies, scans, and clinical exams. We use that information to stage a patient's tumor. This allows us to make appropriate treatment decisions.

SCREENING FOR CANCER

Finding cancer can be difficult. Cancer can spread to other parts of the body, leading to vague symptoms. We want to catch cancer early, before it has a chance to spread. That's the goal of screening, which can help us find cancer before a patient has symptoms.

There are lots of types of screening tests for various types of cancer, depending on a person's age and risk factors. Some tests, such as *mammograms* (breast cancer screening), are recommended by almost everyone. Others, such as *PSA* tests (prostate cancer screening), are controversial.

How do you know whether a screening test is recommended? The US Preventive Services Task Force (USPSTF) is a group of experts that gives grades to screening tests. Grade A means they recommend its use for the general public. Grade D means the task force recommends against using a particular test. Here are some common screening tests:

1. Breast cancer screenings with mammograms, age 50 to 74: Grade B
2. Colon cancer screenings with colonoscopies, age 50 to 75: Grade A
3. Prostate cancer screenings with PSA: Recently changed from Grade D to Grade C
4. Lung cancer screenings with CT scans, age 55 to 80: Grade B
5. Skin cancer screenings with regular skin exams: Grade I—unable to make a recommendation

Screening recommendations are constantly evolving as new information becomes available—as we saw with prostate cancer screenings. Unfortunately, some screening programs are effective but have not been widely adopted (like lung cancer screening) for a variety of reasons. This may be due to a lack of knowledge or resources. For many types of cancers, such as lymphoma, we don't have good screening tests. For other cancers, even if we find them early, we don't have good treatments (like pancreatic cancer). This is frustrating for patients, families, and doctors. Doctors are moving toward more screening and prevention to improve outcomes for patients.

To look at the screening tests available for all sorts of diseases, check out the USPSTF website, listed in the resources at the end of this book.

CANCER OR AN INFECTION?
MAKING SENSE OF A SYMPTOM

Let's go over a common clinical scenario. Bob notices a swollen gland in his neck. He notices slight discomfort with swallowing. He can see inside his mouth in the mirror, and his throat looks slightly red. But he figures he just has a virus and it will go away after a week or two. He has some soup and fluids and rests. His symptoms don't go away, and he goes to the doctor. The doctor checks his neck and is slightly concerned. The doctor writes a prescription for antibiotics, thinking this is bacteria, not a virus, causing the swelling. The gland shrinks down after two weeks. Bob is back to his old self.

Sarah, who works with Bob, also notices a swollen gland in her neck. She has some pain in the area, and she figures it could be a virus. She gives it a week to get better, but it doesn't. The swollen gland just gets bigger. She goes to the same doctor as Bob. The doctor figures there's a strong possibility she caught the same bug, given that she works with Bob. She also has a red throat and some pain in the gland area. She is given the same antibiotics as Bob, but after three weeks, her swollen glands have only gotten bigger.

The doctor orders a biopsy. This involves taking a piece of tissue with a needle and looking at it under a microscope. The biopsy shows she has cancer. Sarah is frustrated, as she wasted one week at home and three to four weeks on antibiotics before the diagnosis of cancer.

It's understandable why Sarah would be mad or distraught. But as you can see, it can be hard to distinguish between these two ailments based on symptoms.

WHY THE GLANDS ARE SWOLLEN

Have you ever had a sore throat with swollen glands?

Those swollen glands are called *lymph nodes*. Lymph nodes are home to the immune system, and they reside all over your body. There are hundreds of them in the neck alone!

When a person is exposed to a virus or bacteria (an invading microbe), the immune system takes that infection to a lymph node. In the lymph node, the white blood cells (immune cells) present the invader to the rest of the immune system. The immune system will then be able to recognize the invader throughout the rest of the body.

Priming of the immune system (exposing it to the bacteria) leads to swelling of the lymph nodes. This is because the immune cells are growing and getting ready to spread throughout the body to hunt down the bacterial invaders. In response to an infection, lymph nodes often seem red, are painful, and may even be hot to the touch.

So what does this have to do with cancer? As we know, cancer cells find organs in which they can grow and flourish. Like the liver or lungs, a lymph node is just another organ where cancer can grow. The organ is like soil for a seed—only this organ is spread all over your body. Many cancers will communicate with the immune cells of the lymph nodes, allowing the cancer cells to take over.

As cancer cells take over the lymph node, the gland swells just like when you're sick from a bacterial infection. But there's one key difference: Cancer cells want to *avoid* the immune system, so they disguise themselves (see chapter 2). Even though cancer grows and fills up a lymph node, the immune system doesn't recognize it's there. There is no immune reaction. It's like the cops don't recognize the bad guys!

Cancer often presents with swollen glands, but the lymph nodes are often less painful than they'd be with an infection (sometimes they're even painless!). Still, the similar symptoms can make it difficult to distinguish between cancer and an infection.

RED FLAGS: SYMPTOMS THAT CALL FOR A CLOSER LOOK

If a patient presents with a painless swollen gland or a painless mass, this is often a red flag for doctors. A *red-flag symptom* is of particular concern to doctors; it's a symptom that's more worrisome than the average symptom we see in clinic.

Red-flag symptoms may include headaches that wake someone up at night, unexplained night sweats or weight loss, and painless swollen masses, among others.

Notice how many of these red-flag symptoms are nonspecific. They might not even signal a cancer diagnosis; they could be caused by something else. A red-flag symptom is only one piece of a puzzle. Having one of these symptoms does *not* mean a person has cancer.

What red flags *do* offer is a key but subtle way to figure out whether a patient has something like Bob (an infection) or Sarah (a cancer). This method isn't perfect. Some patients have both a cancer and an infection. In fact, some cancers make getting an infection more likely. Again, this is why diagnosing cancer is so hard (and why doctors go to school for so long).

STARTING THE WORKUP

Once a patient shows up with a red-flag symptom, doctors pursue a diagnostic workup.

A red flag prompts a doctor to do a more thorough investigation. This includes taking a comprehensive medical history and performing a physical exam. Doctors will often order some basic blood work. These tests look at whether the patient's blood carries enough oxygen (based on the number of red blood cells), is able to fight infections (based on the number of white blood cells, which are the immune cells), and clots correctly (based on the number of platelets).

If doctors suspect a certain type of cancer, they may order a test for tumor markers. *Tumor markers* are proteins that leak out into the blood from tumors. We can then measure the levels of these proteins in the blood.

Most cancer markers are nonspecific. Therefore, they aren't good for screening a population (people) for cancer (see the earlier section on cancer screenings); the markers may be elevated even when there is no cancer. But doctors may use tumor markers to narrow down the possible types of cancer if they suspect a certain cancer in a patient.

GETTING A BIOPSY

We all have normal lumps and bumps in our bodies. These are found everywhere and are a normal part of existence. So how do we tell if something is a normal bump or cancer?

If a doctor identifies a suspicious mass or growth, a *biopsy* is often performed. This means getting a tissue sample using a needle. Why is getting tissue so important? It tells us what we're dealing with—an infection, cancer, or something else.

We have many ways to get the right tissue for a biopsy. If the mass is easy to see and near the skin, a needle can be used to get the tissue without much aid. If a mass is slightly deeper in the body, like in the armpit, an ultrasound probe is often used to guide the needle. Ultrasound uses sound waves to see deeper into tissues. (The same technology is used in pregnancy to see a fetus.) If a mass is deeper in the body, we often use CT (or CAT) scans to help guide the biopsy. A CT scan gives us a 3-D image that allows us to slowly advance a needle to hit the mass.

Many liquid cancers, such as leukemia, don't form a mass we can see for a biopsy. These cancers form from cells that flow through a person's bloodstream. They're found through abnormalities in a person's blood counts when a doctor orders blood tests.

As you may recall, blood cells come from a special material called *bone marrow*, which is found inside large bones, such as the pelvis. For liquid cancers, we often do a bone marrow biopsy. This allows us to better classify a liquid cancer. (See chapter 1 for more information on solid and liquid tumors.)

CAN A BIOPSY SPREAD CANCER?

Many patients are concerned that getting a biopsy will cause a cancer to spread. For the vast majority of cancers, there is *minimal to no risk* of this. (There are a few small exceptions.) In general, this concern should not prevent a biopsy. Doctors need to know what they're dealing with, and the only way to know for sure is to see the tissue under a microscope.

AFTER THE BIOPSY: CANCER UNDER THE MICROSCOPE

The tissue from a biopsy is sent to a pathologist. *Pathologists* are doctors who specialize in diagnosing or identifying tissue. When we ask, "What is that mass?" a pathologist may help solve the mystery.

Pathologists do this by looking at the tissue under a microscope and staining the tumor with special dyes. These dyes stain certain proteins. For example, a woman's breast tumor may stain positive for the *estrogen receptor (ER)* or *progesterone receptor (PR)*—proteins related to female hormones. This staining gives us information about how a cancer may behave and how to treat it.

Pathologists also comment on how abnormal the cells look. They do this by assigning a *grade* to the tumor. Tumor grading is typically on a scale of 1 to 4, but the scale depends on the tumor type. The more abnormal the cells look under a microscope, the higher the grade a pathologist will assign the tumor. In general, high-grade tumors behave more aggressively. They tend to invade normal structures near the tumor and may even spread more often.

One example of the importance of tumor grading is in brain tumors (gliomas). In a low-grade glioma (grade 1) cancer cells appear more like normal brain cells under the microscope. Patients often have a very good prognosis (depending on the exact cancer type). Grade 4 gliomas are brain tumors that look very abnormal under a microscope. These tumors tend to grow rapidly and require aggressive treatment and often have worse long-term outcomes. Certain cancers have special grading systems. For example, in prostate cancer, tumor grading uses the *Gleason score* (see the glossary for details).

Finally, as technology has improved, more and more tumor samples are getting sent out for genetic analysis. *Genetic testing* looks for mutations in the DNA of a cancer. We look to see whether these changes make the cancer vulnerable to a certain treatment. This approach is being used across a range of cancers.

Although patients want answers right away, the results from these tests take a few days. Patients should expect to wait at least two to five days after a biopsy to get results. There are some special genetic tests that may take longer (sometimes weeks). The doctors should discuss that with you and your family before any biopsy or surgery. If there is any question about time frame of results, ask!

After the pathologist checks tissue from the biopsy, they decide what type of cancer it is—if any. Many cancers have fancy scientific names. The details aren't critical, but understanding the general type of cancer is important. Even if you don't remember all the details, I encourage you to write down any fancy scientific names and have them easily available for future doctor visits.

Patients and family members should write down and remember the name of the cancer from the biopsy. (We'll go over a system of organizing this information later on.) Not knowing the type of cancer they have is a mistake many patients make.

Note that it's common for biopsy results to come back inconclusive. This doesn't mean that anyone messed up. Sometimes we need more tissue to make a diagnosis. If this happens, don't be discouraged; discuss with the team what the next steps should be.

THE PURPOSE OF SCANS

If a biopsy confirms cancer, doctors will often order some form of imaging. Sometimes imaging comes before the biopsy; it depends on the type of cancer.

A scan in cancer is often done for one of the three reasons: The first is to check how big the mass is and see whether it's directly invading different organs or structures. The second is to help decide whether we could or should try to cut out the cancer in the operating room. The last is to figure out whether the cancer has spread to other parts of the body.

THE LIMITS OF IMAGING

Although the quality of scans has improved dramatically over the past 20 years, imaging still has significant limitations. With current technology, doctors are unable to see a single cancer cell or even a few million cancer cells on a scan. If we could see every single cancer cell in the body, we would really be onto something big—closer to curing many cancers!

If masses are less than one centimeter (0.4 inches), scans can't reliably separate cancer from normal masses. Imagine plants in a garden: early on, it may be hard to distinguish a weed from the flower you planted!

Once there's a one-centimeter mass, the mass is already somewhere between one hundred million and a billion cells. To give you a sense of scale, the population of Canada is about thirty-seven million, there are about seven to eight billion people on the planet, and there are about two hundred billion stars in our galaxy.

The size and shape of a mass tells us a lot about whether that mass might be cancer. But it takes more than a machine to find cancer. For doctors, having clinical expertise and taking into account the patient's whole picture is critical.

CAN A SCAN TELL IF MY CANCER TREATMENT IS WORKING?

For the majority of patients, we don't order scans during cancer treatment. There are two main reasons: The first is our inability to see single cancer cells on scans. If cancer cells are dying, we won't be able to see it until millions of cells have died. The second reason is the lag time between the death of the cancer cells and what we see on a scan. It can take weeks for a mass to disappear, even if all the cells have died. This is because it can take that long for the body to remove the dead cells and repair the region.

Most of the time, it isn't helpful to get a scan during cancer treatment. Often, scans during treatment only make patients and families anxious. (Of course, there are exceptions. We often get PET/CT scans when treating lymphomas.)

CHOOSING THE RIGHT SCAN

The type of scan depends on the part of the body we want to look at. It also depends on the type of cancer. The most commonly ordered scans include CT scans (also known as CAT scans), MRI scans, bone scans, and PET/CT scans.

CT scans are helpful for seeing the details of organs, lymph nodes, and other parts of the body very clearly. These scans are fast and are often easy for patients to tolerate. CT scans use X-rays to look inside the body.

An *MRI* uses magnetic fields to help us peer inside a person. MRIs are best at looking at soft tissues—like the normal folds of the brain or the soft tissue of the arm or leg. Downsides of an MRI include time and patient comfort. These scans can take anywhere from a half hour to more than an hour. The patients are put into small tubes, and some people describe them as claustrophobic and loud.

Nuclear-medicine tests use a radioactive substance or material, called a *tracer*, that is placed in the body. If an area of the body takes up too much or too little tracer, it may imply there's a cancer or other problem. Common nuclear-medicine tests include *bone scans* and PET/CT scans.

The use of PET/CT is common across a variety of cancers. Notice the name *PET/CT.* When you get a PET scan, you also get a CT scan—two for one!

PET/CT: TEAMING UP TO FIND
HIGH SUGAR CONSUMPTION

Preparing for PET/CT scans involves injecting a labeled sugar that's taken up by the body; we can then see that sugar on a scanner. Cancer cells use up lots of sugar quickly and inefficiently (remember the *Warburg effect*), so we can see cancer cells "light up" on PET/CT scans.

The lighting up of a region in PET is called *activity*. The activity indicates how much sugar a part of the body has taken up, which gives the region a glow. The greater the glow, the faster the cells are using sugar, and the more of them there are. Sounds like cancer, right?

The PET image we get is grainy. This makes it hard to determine exactly where the activity is. To help pinpoint the area, we get a CT scan the same day. That's why we get a PET and CT together—to see the activity and help localize it.

So why wouldn't we just use PET/CT for everything? A PET depends on cells taking up labeled sugar. The cancer cells want to use sugar because they're trying to overtake the rest of the body, like weeds in a garden. They need the energy to keep things moving. But there are also normal fast-growing cells that take up sugar—say, cells of the immune system. Immune system cells take up a lot of sugar to fight off invaders or even cancer! It's often hard to tell inflammation from cancer on a scan.

Furthermore, not all cancer cells reliably take up the labeled sugar. A PET/CT scan is good for seeing some cancers but bad for others.

PET/CT scans are also of limited use in parts of the body that use lots of sugar normally, like the brain. The brain is always working hard and taking in lots of sugar. This makes it hard to see any cancer that might have gone to the brain.

Finally, you may remember the magical one-centimeter size in scans. PET/CT scans are no different! These scans have limited resolution; they can't see a single cancer cell. Masses that aren't big enough don't show up in the scans.

PUTTING TOGETHER THE CLUES

Doctors gather all this information to determine the diagnosis (the type of cancer seen under the microscope) and the stage of the cancer. These two things have the biggest influence on how to move forward with care.

We use the diagnosis, clinical examination, and the scans we obtained to provide a clinical stage.

TNM: A SECRET LANGUAGE FOR STAGES OF CANCER

Staging depends on the type of cancer, but we generally define staging in two areas: clinical versus pathological stage. This is often confusing to patients.

Clinical stage is determined using information from a physical exam and scans. A *pathological stage* is determined after surgery (we'll talk about pathological stage in chapter 6, where we discuss surgery).

So if you've had a biopsy, isn't your stage a pathological stage? No! The biopsy just helps confirm what type of cancer a person has. The pathological stage is classified after a surgical procedure on the cancer—that is, after removing the mass or lymph nodes.

As part of a first diagnosis, a patient gets a clinical stage. The clinical stage is broken up into three parts: T (tumor), N (lymph nodes), and M (metastasis). This is called the *TNM staging system*, and it's used across a range of cancers. The criteria vary depending on the cancer type, but here are the general principles:

- T considers the size of the tumor.
- N looks at the number of lymph nodes into which the cancer has spread (see chapter 2 for more on lymph nodes).
- M considers whether the cancer has spread, or *metastasized*, to other organs (liver, lungs, and so on).

Each one of these groups gets a number. For example, if a woman has a 2.5-centimeter mass in the breast and one lymph node is involved, her stage is T2N1M0.

Most often, when doctors talk about cancer with patients, we do not discuss the TNM. Doctors often only discuss the final stage or group the patient falls into, which you'll read about in the next section.

STAGING: GROUPING PATIENTS

The final steps in staging a cancer use the TNM language to place a patient into a group—also known as the final *stage*. The woman in our scenario with a T2N1M0 breast cancer would be given a Stage II classification. Stages help us predict how the cancer will behave and what the potential outcome for the patient may be.

Just like TNM varies across different cancers, so do staging groups. Staging often goes from I to IV (or 1 to 4, using Roman numerals). Stage I means the cancer is local (it's a small cancer with no signs of spread to other parts of the body). On the other hand, Stage IV often implies the cancer has spread to other parts of the body.

This does *not* mean that Stage IV is always bad or incurable. There are some patients with Stage IV cancers that still may be cured of their cancer (see chapter 9 on the gray zone). Patients need to talk to their doctors to understand what a stage means in the context of a specific cancer.

BRINGING IT ALL TOGETHER

Patients need to understand the name of their type of cancer so they can communicate with doctors and other clinicians. To keep track of information, write down the name of the cancer (diagnosis) and the stage. This allows patients to speak up for themselves in regard to their health and better understand their cancer. Not knowing the diagnosis or stage is a mistake many patients make.

Mistake #1: Not knowing the name and stage of their cancer

The diagnosis, grade, and stage give doctors a sense of how a cancer may behave. This helps determine how to balance treatments. We can then put together a medical and emotional support team to help the patient decide how to move forward. We'll talk about putting these teams together in the upcoming chapters.

Chapter Four

The Emotional Toll of Cancer

Receiving a cancer diagnosis is life changing. When people hear the words *You have cancer*, their minds turn off. Those words may be the only thing they take away from the doctor's appointment. There's a whirlwind of emotions, and it can be hard to take everything in. Because processing the information is so hard, patients should write down their questions, concerns, emotions, and everything in between.

Patients, families, and doctors sometimes overlook the emotional difficulties that arise when dealing with a cancer diagnosis. Remember that you're not alone in your journey: family, friends, doctors, nurses, support groups, and social workers are all there for you. In this chapter, we discuss the emotional aspects of a cancer diagnosis and where you can go for help.

WHY YOU WANT AN EMOTIONAL SUPPORT TEAM

What's the right emotional response to hearing you have cancer?

There is no "right" response.
Crying is normal.
Anger is normal.
Yelling is normal.
Denial is normal.
Many people feel a loss of control over their lives.

Remember, a person's emotions are *not* the enemy in this situation. Patients need to work through these emotions. To do so, a patient should form an emotional support team made up of family, friends, neighbors, counselors, and others.

Being honest with the emotional support team—whoever that may include—can help alleviate fears, worries, doubts, and other painful emotions. Whether you're a patient, a family member, or a close friend, don't be afraid to seek help.

PICKING THE PROS AS PART OF THE TEAM

Seeking out an emotional support team is helpful for many cancer patients. The professional part of this team can include survivorship groups, counselors, social workers, psychologists, and psychiatrists.

In fact, there are psychologists and psychiatrists who specialize in working with patients with cancer. This is because depression and anxiety are common responses to a cancer diagnosis. It can be hard to deal with this on your own.

I always urge patients and families to seek help early and often. Many cancer patients and families benefit from talk therapy, medications (such as antidepressants or antianxiety medications), and other treatments these providers may offer.

Seeking psychological help is a normal part of dealing with cancer. The cancer center working with the patient can help direct you to the resources available inside or outside the center.

DID I BRING THIS ON MYSELF? THE BLAME GAME

Guilt is a common emotion that arises upon receiving a cancer diagnosis. Some people feel as if they brought the cancer on themselves because of habits such as smoking or drinking. Addictions such as drug use, smoking, or alcoholism are real medical problems that can be hard to treat.

I want to stress that *no one deserves cancer*.

Coping with cancer is a heartbreaking process, and the person diagnosed shouldn't be made to feel guilty. Instead, they should focus on growing their medical and emotional support teams and pursuing their passions. Of course, quitting those bad habits may be helpful in the long term (see chapter 12, on nutrition and lifestyle, for help).

GET ORGANIZED: REGAINING A FEELING OF CONTROL

We need to take a step-by-step approach to cancer and a person's emotional reaction to it. To start, remember mistake #1: not knowing the diagnosis and stage of cancer. To help keep information straight, make a treatment binder that has all the documents regarding diagnosis, treatment, and medical information.

In this binder, break information into groups: Medication List, Medical Appointments, Diagnosis, Pathology Reports, Scan Reports, Side Effects, and Other. I prefer a three-ring binder; you can then hole-punch papers to organize information into sections. This may help you bring order from the chaos.

Organization helps bring back a feeling of control over everything that is happening, which helps decrease the anxiety many patients feel. But if you or family members can't work on this binder right away, don't feel like you have to.

When you feel ready, make a system that works for you to stay organized. There are many premade organization systems out there. Find whatever works. I talk more about maintaining patient information in the next chapter, on determining cancer treatment.

FASTER IS NOT BETTER: ALLOWING TIME TO FORMULATE A TREATMENT PLAN

When someone finds out they have cancer, we doctors may need more information (another scan or biopsy) before we decide on treatment. Many patients have trouble waiting. They push doctors and nurses to get started with treatment right away.

Commonly, I hear patients say, "Doc, I have cancer. Don't you get it? I want to get started with my treatment today." I can understand and sympathize with these feelings, both the stress and the anxiety.

There is one principle of cancer care I always share with my patients:

A comprehensive cancer plan, with all the needed clinical information, is always better than a fast treatment plan.

Getting started quickly can lead us down the wrong road. If this happens, it can affect the outcome of treatment. Thus we should get all the clinical information before making a decision on treatment.

This delay can lead the patient to feel frustrated and even angry. Recognize these feelings, and know that everyone is working hard to help the patient deal with the cancer. Always advocate for the best care, but try to keep in mind that the doctors want to get started with the treatment too; we just want to make sure we have all the information we need first. This sometimes means fighting with insurance companies to get another scan, biopsy, or genetic test.

DON'T QUIT YOUR DAY JOB AND MOVE TO THE BAHAMAS . . . YET

After a diagnosis of cancer, patients often rush to make big life decisions or changes. Some patients feel the need to sell their house, move, change jobs, or even file for divorce.

Some patients are trying to escape their current life. Others are searching for the life they wish they'd lived.

I urge patients to *not* make big financial or personal decisions soon after a diagnosis of cancer. Let the news settle. Make time to talk to family and friends about fear, anxiety, and uncertainty. Discuss everything going on with your emotional support team, and seek help and encouragement.

"ETERNITY IS IN LOVE WITH THE CREATIONS OF TIME": PURSUING YOUR PASSIONS

Cancer can make clear what is most essential to each of us: family, painting, playing the violin, traveling the world, writing a book, and so much more.

As a result, patients tend to react in one of two ways to a cancer diagnosis. Some patients use this turn of events to hold even closer the things they value. Other patients push the things they care about most as far away as possible. They desire to shield loved ones from a life they fear is doomed.

Many people make rash decisions in trying to get away from their families, hoping to spare them the pain of the diagnosis, treatment, and potential outcomes. It is in trying to protect those they love in this way, ironically, that they often hurt their loved ones the most. Family and friends only wish to be there with the patient through this journey. Rather, patients should use the cancer diagnosis to bring loved ones closer. I also urge patients with cancer to pursue dreams and passions, no matter what stage of cancer they're in.

But didn't I just say not to make major life changes or choices after a diagnosis? You're right. I wouldn't make those major changes right after a diagnosis. But after a treatment is agreed upon, patients can start thinking about making their dreams and passions a reality. Dreams and passions are a critical part of who we are. (So feel free to start planning that trip to the Bahamas.)

My favorite quotation comes from poet William Blake on the subject of creation: "Eternity is in love with the creations of time." This creation could include traveling the world, writing your book, or seeing the Chicago Cubs play in Wrigley Field. A goal or dream gives you something to look forward to and allows you to pursue what's most essential in your life. I urge patients to discuss dreams and passions openly with their medical and emotional support teams.

SEEKING SPIRITUAL SUPPORT

Even if you aren't religious, this next section is worth a read.

Please know that you don't need a religious affiliation to take advantage of spiritual support. Chaplains are spiritually trained practitioners who help patients in all stages of illness. They are well versed in a variety of religious practices. They may also connect patients to a spiritual leader or pray with them directly.

Some people are afraid to ask for spiritual support after a cancer diagnosis. They don't want to bother the rabbi or priest. But I've found that the spiritual leaders of communities love being involved in the care of patients. For patients, friends, and family, getting help is just a matter of reaching out.

If a patient has a connection with a religion but doesn't have a spiritual leader, doctors can connect them to chaplain services. Do not ignore the spiritual side of a cancer diagnosis. A spiritual guide can be part of an emotional support team.

Many providers forget about this aspect of care; go ahead and ask about it! We're always happy to help you find your way.

PREPARING FOR THE JOURNEY OF CANCER

Cancer is a journey. Doctors, nurses, social workers, religious leaders, and spouses all go through this journey with the patient—no matter where it leads. Know that whether you're the patient, a spouse, another family member, or a friend, you aren't alone on this journey.

Patients should seek out emotional and spiritual help early in this process. Not doing so is the second common mistake patients make:

Mistake #2: Not seeking emotional and religious support early

Chapter Five

Deciding on Goals and Treatment

We now have all the diagnostic information we need, and an emotional support team is in place. We now need to decide how to move forward with treatment.

Doctors should spell out the goal of cancer treatment for each patient. By *goal* I mean that the treatment should have one of two intentions:

1. *Curative intent*: This means we're trying to cure the cancer.
2. *Palliative intent*: This means we're managing pain and the effects of the cancer on life. The goal of treatment is not to cure the cancer but to maintain the patient's life for as long as we can with as much quality as possible.

Stating the goal of treatment helps patients understand where treatment is going and what they can expect. As with all things in life, there is often a gray zone between curative and palliative intent, but it's helpful to have a starting point. Of particular importance is the gray zone of *oligometastatic* patients (see the glossary and chapter 9) and the evolving treatments for this particular group. We will review this in detail later on. In regard to reviewing the goals of care, you can find a doctor's appointment cheat sheet to help identify goals of care at stephenrosenbergmd.com.

This chapter is the most significant in the book, as we'll also go over three common mistakes in this chapter.

LOOKING AT DAY-TO-DAY PERFORMANCE

To decide on the goals of care, many factors are taken into account. This includes the type of cancer, the stage of the cancer, and the performance status of the patient. In past chapters, we have talked about cancer types (liquid versus solid) and cancer stages. We'll focus this discussion on performance status.

Have you ever walked into a room and said, "That person doesn't look well"? What are you measuring when you say that?

A person may look ashen or thin, indicating they aren't eating or have poor nutrition. They may be too weak to get out of bed, meaning their muscles aren't working well.

Performance status aims to quantify how a person is functioning globally, in all aspects of their lives. Is a person able to get out of bed and dress themselves? Are they able to make their own food and feed themselves?

Overall, determining performance status means trying to figure out how much of a person's daily activities they can do on their own. Cancer doctors obsess over performance status.

Across a range of studies, performance status is the biggest predictor of how people will do with treatment. It predicts life expectancy and a patient's ability to tolerate treatments.

If someone has a bad performance status, that patient will likely have a poor outcome, regardless of treatment. For example, a patient who is morbidly obese and can't get out of bed is unlikely to tolerate cancer treatment. Even if they do tolerate treatment, there's a reasonable probability they'll die of something other than cancer (such as a blood clot, stroke, or heart attack). Compare that to a patient who is a marathon runner in their early 30s. They'll likely be better able to tolerate aggressive chemotherapy, surgery, and radiation.

QUALITY VERSUS QUANTITY OF LIFE
(SPOILER: BOTH ARE IMPORTANT!)

Regardless of the intention of treatment—curative or palliative—all cancer doctors focus on two things for patients when deciding on treatment: the quality and quantity of life.

Both have to be a consideration. If we give a patient an extra month of life but they can't talk or get out of bed, did we help them? Considering both of these factors allows us to weigh the risks and benefits of any treatment.

We know cancer is sneaky. Hitting cancer with many types of treatments (surgery, chemotherapy, immunotherapy, etc.) makes it less likely that the cancer will be resistant to therapy. The downside is that the more types of treatment we use, the more toxic the treatment. We also know that if a treatment is too toxic, patients won't finish it. If a patient gets only partway through a treatment, it's less likely to help them.

Some side effects are lasting, so we also want to consider the quality of life after cancer. For example, for a patient who wants to have a family, we'll want to look at how a potential treatment may affect fertility. (You'll read about fertility and sexuality in chapter 12.)

THE NUMBER ONE TENET OF ONCOLOGY: DO NO MORE THAN YOU HAVE TO

Here's a tenet in cancer treatment that I think is critical: The best medicine is doing as much *nothing* as possible. (I attribute this idea to Samuel Shem [the pen name for Stephen Bergman], an author and psychiatrist.)

Giving chemotherapy, radiation, or some other form of treatment isn't always in the best interests of the patient. This can be hard to hear. When doctors take into account all the factors (diagnosis, stage, and performance status), we have to figure out whether treatment will help the patient.

For some patients, hospice care is helpful (and is a form of treatment!). *Hospice care* is end-of-life care that supports the patient and loved ones through advanced illness. This kind of care can be administered at home or in a facility. We'll discuss hospice care in greater detail in chapter 11.

BUILDING THE TREATMENT TEAM

The first doctor a patient with cancer is referred to is often a surgeon or medical oncologist (chemotherapy doctor). Regardless of which doctor a person sees first, the patient will work with that first doctor to build a medical team: a group of experts who will help treat their cancer.

Who makes up the medical team depends on the goals of care, the type of cancer, and the performance status of the patient. Many other people are essential parts of the medical team (such as nurses and physical therapists), but I'm focusing this discussion on the people who make medical decisions on cancer treatment.

If a patient has a liquid tumor, the treatment team typically consists of a medical oncologist (a doctor who prescribes chemotherapy and immunotherapy) and a radiation oncologist (a doctor who prescribes radiation). We'll go over chemotherapy, radiation therapy, and immunotherapy in upcoming chapters.

If a patient has a solid tumor, the treatment team often consists of a medical oncologist, a radiation oncologist, and a surgeon. The type of surgeon depends on which part of the body the cancer is found in. Some surgeons specialize in cancers of the head and neck (ear, nose, and throat—or ENT—surgeons, also known as *otolaryngologists*), the bowels (colorectal surgeons), or other parts of the body.

There's a notable exception to the treatment team in gynecological cancers (cancers of the ovaries, uterus, or female reproductive tract). There are GYN oncologists who both perform surgery *and* give chemotherapy. They're unique in the oncology system.

THE FORGOTTEN TEAMMATES: PALLIATIVE CARE PROVIDERS

As treatment plans evolve, one team member is often forgotten: the palliative care doctor. I devote chapter 11 to palliative care and hospice, but I wanted to touch on this type of care here first.

Palliative care doctors specialize in relieving pain and other symptoms of life-threatening illnesses such as cancer. They can go above and beyond to help treat both the physical aspects and the emotional strain of cancer.

Data shows that early involvement in palliative care may improve outcomes for patients. Many doctors forget to refer patients to palliative care, so it may be something to ask about. Palliative care providers should be part of a medical team.

THE TUMOR BOARD: MURKY WATERS ARE DANGEROUS, SO LOAD THE BOAT

Sometimes determining which treatment course to follow is unclear. Many patient cases don't fit neatly into a textbook answer. When that happens, doctors often present a patient's case at a tumor board.

In a *tumor board*, a group of doctors from different specialties (medical oncology, radiation oncology, surgery, etc.) meet to discuss patients who have a particular type of cancer, such as breast or lung cancer. The doctors check scans, pathology, and everything else about the patient to try to agree on a treatment plan. Doctors then relay that information back to the patient and family.

ADVOCATE FOR THE TEAM: KEEPING EVERYONE IN THE LOOP

It's essential that everyone in the treatment team agree on the plan. Always try to clear up confusing points before the end of a doctor's appointment. Doctors can forget to explain aspects of care that seem obvious to them but are new to you, so go ahead and ask for explanations. There's no such thing as a stupid question.

Doctors are human too. They sometimes forget to make referrals to other members of a treatment team. If you meet with a surgeon, does the surgeon need to refer you to a medical oncologist or a radiation oncologist? If you meet with a medical oncologist, do they need to refer you to a radiation oncologist or a surgeon? Ask away! There is a cheat sheet to help ensure you get appropriate referrals at stephenrosenbergmd.com/.

GET ORGANIZED: KNOW THE NAME AND STAGE OF THE CANCER

No matter which of the doctors a patient meets with first, there are a few points to take away from early conversations: What is the diagnosis? What is the stage of the cancer? (Remember mistake #1 in chapter 3.)

Trying to keep this information organized is key. A blank sheet of paper will do, but as noted before take a look at stephenrosenbergmd.com for some free templates to bring to the doctor's office.

Making a treatment binder can help you deal with information over-load (see chapter 4 for details). As a patient moves between doctor's appointments, each doctor will have their own handouts and informa-tional packets. I prefer to put them in a three-ring binder to keep all the information together. Whatever system works for you or the patient is the one to stick with.

SHOULD FAMILY AND FRIENDS COME TO APPOINTMENTS?

Regarding doctor's appointments, family and friends must respect the wishes of the patient (whether that's you or someone you care about). Some people think that bringing everyone in the family to the doctor's appointment is the way to go. I find this forces many clinic visits to be more superficial. A grandfather doesn't want to talk about death or dying with his fifteen-year-old grandson in the room.

I tell families that, ideally, anywhere from one to five people should go with a patient to an appointment. Make sure everyone is old enough to handle hard discussions. It is key that the patient feels comfortable having those discussions with the people present.

ASK QUESTIONS

Formally discuss the goals of care during early appointments. The goal of any treatment should be defined as "curative" or "palliative." (But realize there may be some overlap. Real life is often not so black and white.) When talking with the medical team about added scans or pro-cedures, find out whether they're necessary. What are the risks and benefits?

You'll also want to consider long-term plans. When deciding on treatment, be open with the medical team, your partners, and your family members regarding wishes for family planning.

There is so much information to take in during these early appoint-ments; it's nearly impossible to keep it all straight. To keep organized, write things down (use the binder), including any questions anyone has. It's extremely helpful to have a few people come to the appointment, with one person as the designated recorder. The other people at the appointment are there to carefully listen and try to take in what the doctors are saying. Patients and families should be sure to organize this information.

Everyone should leave the doctor's appointments with a clear appreciation of the plan, the goals, and the next steps. Again, don't be afraid to ask questions! This is the next common mistake patients make:

Mistake #3: Being afraid to ask questions

This includes clarifications on treatment, plans, and prognosis. Staying quiet can lead to a lack of understanding of the goals of treatment.

GETTING SURVIVAL ESTIMATES: AM I AVERAGE?

Some patients like to hear about outcomes—for example, the average survival rate of patients with a particular cancer at five or ten years. If a patient has a certain type of brain tumor, that person may want to know the average length of survival. This can help them with family planning and financial issues. It may also help them decide how to spend their time (see chapter 4 on the emotional impact cancer can have).

But no person is a number. An average is just that—an average. There are no absolutes.

Some people will live shorter than the average, but others will live longer. Because of this, some patients don't want to hear about averages or other such numbers. Whatever works for the patient should be the focus. Patients need to communicate with doctors what they want to hear.

Sometimes patients and families want to hear about different things. If a family member wants to hear about statistics or patient averages but the patient doesn't, consider arranging separate conversations. The doctor can discuss additional information with the family as long as the patient consents to it.

INVITE SECOND OPINIONS: THE ART OF MEDICINE

Medicine is an art and a science. If medicine were just a science, it would be much easier to practice. Interpretation of data and judgment are key to the practice of medicine which leads to different opinions on treatment. There are often many correct approaches for addressing any one given problem (or cancer). Many patients or families are fearful to ask for a second opinion because they don't want to hurt the doctor's feelings.

Most doctors welcome a second opinion. Maybe another doctor has a new clinical trial your doctor is unaware of. You never know. Asking for a second opinion is an aspect of being active in a patient's care and can help reassure family and friends. This is another common mistake patients make:

Mistake #4: Being afraid to ask for a second opinion

Remember, more treatment isn't always better. I would stress that the current US health care system gives doctors incentives to perform treatments on patients. For example, doctors get paid to give chemotherapy, radiation, and so on. So if four doctors recommend against chemotherapy, there still may be a fifth who would offer it. If you look hard enough, you'll find someone to administer treatment *whether or not it's in the best interests of the patient*. The doctors whom other doctors most respect are those who know when to treat and when *not* to treat.

GETTING MORE INFORMATION: ACCESS TO DOCTORS' RESOURCES

When a patient meets with a cancer doctor, the doctor takes into account the patient's diagnosis (cancer type), stage (including any genetic tests), and performance status. Using all this information, doctors decide on a treatment regimen.

We base this decision on multiple sources, such as evidence from clinical trials and reports from the scientific literature. We doctors also use our individual training and the resources put together by national organizations. Two of these resources are worth mentioning:

- *NCCN*: The National Comprehensive Cancer Network uses scientific evidence and expert opinion to put together trustworthy guidelines on how to treat various cancers. You can access these guidelines for free if you make an account (see the link in the resources at the end of the book). Keep in mind that the language in clinical guidelines can be hard to understand, as they are written for doctors. NCCN also makes excellent resources for patients that are less detailed.

- *UpToDate*: This subscription-based website is used by doctors all over the world. It's a living, breathing textbook that has the most up-to-date medical information on many topics. If you want trustworthy information or further reading, this is an excellent site, but, again, it's written for doctors. You may be able to access UpToDate for free at some university libraries.

END-OF-LIFE DECISIONS

More people than ever are surviving after a cancer diagnosis. Many people go on to live long, healthy lives after cancer. Regardless, a diagnosis of cancer should be used as an opportunity to discuss health care issues within a family.

Family and friends need to understand what a patient's wishes are for end-of-life care. The person dealing with cancer should designate who will make health care decisions for them if they can't make decisions themselves; this stand-in is known as a *health care proxy*.

The emotional support team and spiritual guides (see chapter 4) may help a patient determine their end-of-life wishes. It's critical to convey those wishes to the medical doctors so we may honor them.

It's also extremely helpful if the family knows about a loved one's finances before they pass away or get very ill. Many patients fail to think about these things. Finances are best dealt with when a person is well rather than very sick.

A patient should also meet with a financial advisor, lawyer, and other trusted confidantes to make sure a will is set up properly. This can prevent years of hardship for families after a patient has passed away. Social workers can also help refer you to professionals to work out these issues.

These preparations are excellent things to keep in mind, whether you have cancer or not. Avoiding end-of-life and financial issues is another common mistake patients make:

Mistake #5: Not discussing finances, wills, health care proxies, and other end-of-life issues with family, doctors, and friends before or soon after a diagnosis, regardless of cancer stage or potential outcomes

Chapter 5

DOING OUR BEST

In cancer, as in life, there are no guarantees. Doctors do the best they can with the information and tools available. We use our skills and knowledge to help patients and families make informed decisions. Patients, families, friends, and neighbors should also help speak up for the patient to make sure they're getting everything they need.

In the upcoming chapters, we'll break down the types of treatment that may be used to combat cancer.

Chapter Six

Surgery

Surgery was one of the first types of treatment for cancer, and techniques keep improving.

Surgery plays a major role in treatment for many patients, making a surgeon a critical part of the cancer treatment team. Still, patients should recognize that surgery might not help everyone. (Notable exceptions include patients with liquid cancers, such as leukemia, that don't have a mass to cut out.)

Decisions on surgery should be made with a patient's medical team, with the treatment's intent (cure or palliative) in mind. The diagnosis, cancer stage, and treatment goals will determine whether chemotherapy and radiation should be given before or after surgery.

MORE SURGERY IS NOT BETTER

A common feeling patients have when they're diagnosed with cancer is that they just want the cancer out. But *more surgery* does not mean better outcomes. The trend in medicine has been to try less-radical surgeries to limit side effects and better support quality of life.

If we cut out cancer, why would it come back? There are many reasons. Let's go back to the weed analogy. First, even though a weed is removed, it may have left seeds nearby, allowing a new weed to grow. In the case of cancer, a few cancer cells escaping from the main tumor is basically like a seed. This can allow the cancer to regrow in another area nearby. Second, if you've ever worked in a garden, you

45

know you need to remove a weed by its roots to get rid of it. In the same way, if we don't get rid of all the cancer cells, there's a high chance the tumor will grow back in the same place.

The key to a successful surgery is to do everything reasonable to remove cancer in its entirety. So why not do more radical surgery? Why not remove the whole plot of soil from the garden, taking the weeds with it? This could help make sure the weeds don't come back. But if seeds have already drifted on the wind to another area of the garden, we've significantly damaged the garden and the weeds are still present, now in a new place.

The aggressive removal of tumors and tissues was tried in the early twentieth century. The surgery for breast cancer was a *radical mastectomy*, which involved removing the breast, the underlying muscle, and most of the lymph nodes in the armpit. Although the surgery was disfiguring, it was the standard treatment up until the 1970s. Now, studies have shown that less tissue can be taken out with the same outcomes and fewer side effects. This type of surgery is called a *modified mastectomy*. In surgery, *more* does not always equal *better*.

As I mentioned, surgery is often a central part of cancer care, but it's only one pillar in the overall treatment.

CHEMOTHERAPY AND RADIATION BEFORE OR AFTER SURGERY? OR EVER?

Cancer doesn't exist as a smooth, round ball. Like a weed, the tumor extends roots into the normal tissue it invades. We know that in order to prevent the cancer from coming back, we need to remove all the roots as well.

No matter how good surgeons are, when removing a cancer, they can't see cells without a microscope in the operating room. That's why surgeons try to take some normal-appearing tissue from around the tumor during surgery. This extra tissue is the definition of a *surgical margin*.

When a surgeon says the margins "are clean," it means there's a rim of healthy tissue that's free of cancer surrounding the tumor. This implies that most of the cancer was likely taken out. The roots have been removed!

As mentioned, surgeons can't see the cells (or the roots of the tumor) during surgery. There's always the possibility that some cancer cells will be left behind. If they're left in the body and are allowed to grow, they'll form a new mass. This is called a *local recurrence* of a cancer.

Giving radiation or chemotherapy before surgery can cause the cancer to shrink and may destroy those roots. Shrinking the mass can help a surgeon get a rim of normal-appearing tissue and more easily remove the tumor. This may decrease the chances a cancer will come back.

By giving chemotherapy or radiation up front, doctors also get a sense of how a cancer will respond to treatment. In some instances, this lets us better predict how the cancer will behave.

This approach doesn't work with all cancers. Some tumor cells won't respond to chemotherapy or radiation. For some tumors, a delay in surgery may lead to a worse outcome. The patient should discuss the order of treatments with the medical team.

Patients and families should also realize that not every cancer needs chemotherapy or radiation after surgery. Sometimes surgery is all that's needed!

WAIT—WHAT TYPE OF DOCTOR?

Surgeons in the realm of cancer tend to specialize. Lots of data suggests that in doing one thing over and over again, a person becomes an expert. Therefore, it makes sense for surgeons to specialize in certain operations or parts of the body.

For example, an otolaryngologist (also called an ENT—ear, nose, and throat doctor) will do surgeries of the head and neck. Separately trained specialists perform breast cancer surgeries. Another example of a specialist is a gynecologic oncologist, who does operations related to the female reproductive tract.

The patient and family should be comfortable with the surgeon. Patients should also research whether the surgeon has the proper experience with the type of surgery in question.

SCALPEL, PLEASE: TYPES OF SURGERY

There are many ways to approach surgery, depending on the location of the cancer in the body. Here are some terms patients often hear when discussing their upcoming surgeries with their cancer care team:

- *Open surgery*: This is a traditional surgery. An incision is made in order to see the tumor, insert instruments, and remove the mass.
- *Nerve-sparing surgery*: The idea is to perform an operation that leaves the nerves controlling that part of the body intact.
- *Laparoscopic (minimally invasive) surgery*: This often involves a much smaller incision to reduce trauma to the body and reduce blood loss. Small incisions are made (0.5 to 2.0 centimeters). This surgery uses a *laparoscope*, which is a camera that allows doctors to see that area of the body.
- *Robotic surgery*: Many patients hear of robotic surgery. One system is named the *da Vinci Surgical System* (this is just a type of machine used). Robotic surgery is a type of minimally invasive surgery. Robotic arms, controlled by the surgeon, can help do delicate tasks in an operation and allow for small incisions. Robotic surgery may lead to less blood loss, less pain, and swifter recovery.

CONSTRUCTION ON THE IMMUNE-SYSTEM HIGHWAY: ASSESSING LYMPH NODES

Earlier we noted that cancer can spread to lymh nodes. Remember, swelling of the lymph nodes may be a sign a cancer is spreading (see chapter 3). It's hard to discern whether a lymph node has cancer if the mass is less than one centimeter in size.

Tumor cells often drain to nearby lymph node regions, which can be another environment for the cells to divide and thrive in. To assess nearby lymph nodes and prevent cancer from spreading further, old surgical techniques used to call for taking out any lymph nodes that were downstream from a cancer. This involves taking out a lot of lymph nodes—10 to 30 of them. This surgery is called a *complete lymph node dissection*, and it comes with the risk of significant side effects.

Removing lymph nodes disrupts the natural flow of fluid through the body. The more lymph nodes removed, the more radical the disruption. This can lead to significant swelling of an arm or leg or impair the function of a body part (*lymphedema*—see glossary).

We now better recognize how cancer cells move to lymph nodes. We use that knowledge to predict how cancer will spread.

THE FIRST STOP: SENTINEL LYMPH NODES

For many cancers, we look for the *sentinel lymph nodes* at the time of surgery. This is the first group of lymph nodes the cancer cells may drain to. This is like the first stop of a train on a track. If we remove the first-stop lymph nodes and there's no cancer there, it's unlikely cancer has spread beyond that point. This can allow us to avoid taking out many lymph nodes, which would lead to significant side effects. In fact, removing sentinel lymph nodes has been used in successfully treating breast cancer and a host of other cancers.

How do we find sentinel lymph nodes? During surgery, a surgeon injects a dye containing a radioactive tracer into the tumor. The dye drains to the first-stop lymph nodes, turning them blue. The surgeon uses a special scanner in the operating room to confirm the radioactive tracer is in that lymph node. Often, these sentinel lymph nodes consist of one to three lymph nodes, which are then taken out as a group.

If cancer is found in this first group of lymph nodes, patients may need additional surgery. This means going on to a complete lymph node dissection (taking out more lymph nodes). However, removing more isn't always required. It depends on the clinical scenario. Patients need to discuss the next steps with their surgeon, depending on the results of the sentinel lymph node test.

The sentinel lymph node test doesn't work well for all cancer types. You can discuss the decision to look for sentinel lymph nodes with your surgeon.

GOING TO SLEEP: UNDERSTANDING ANESTHESIA

A patient will meet with the surgeon and an anesthesia team before an operation. Some tests are done to make sure a patient is healthy enough for an operation. These tests are often aimed at assessing the patient's heart and lung function.

The goal of most cancer surgeries is to remove the entire tumor (with that clear margin). There should always be a thorough discussion of the risks and benefits of surgery before a patient undergoes an operation.

Many patients forget to ask some practical questions of the surgical and anesthesia teams: How long will the operation take? What type of anesthesia will be used? Who do we talk to for updates during the operation? How many days in the hospital do we anticipate?

There are many different approaches to giving anesthesia during a cancer operation. Anesthesia may include a *local* injection, which involves numbing a specific area of the body. Surgery often involves both local and *general anesthesia*, which means getting put to sleep and having a breathing tube placed.

If you've had a bad interaction with anesthesia, let the anesthesia team and surgeon know. It's also vital to make sure that the anesthesiologist has an up-to-date list of all medications you're taking and allergies you have.

DURING THE OPERATION

For many family members and friends, knowing how long an operation will take gives them some sense of control.

Before surgery begins, find out whom family and friends can ask for updates during the procedure. Getting updates can help calm fears and nerves during the operation. If an operation runs long, that does *not* mean something is wrong.

The more knowledge a patient and loved ones have about an operation, the better prepared they'll be to handle any bumps in the road.

AFTER THE OPERATION

The surgeon will often come talk to the family or friends to inform them how the surgery went and offer any updates. After surgery, some patients may be allowed to go home the same day. Other patients will stay in the hospital for a number of days, depending on the type of surgery.

Patients must be able to perform self-care before they're allowed to go home from the hospital. This includes being able to eat or drink, use the bathroom, and walk steps that may be at home. A patient's pain should be at the point of requiring only pills (no IV-administered medications) before leaving the hospital.

Walking soon after surgery (as allowed by the doctors) helps prevent clots from developing, which can be deadly, and pneumonia. Family and doctors should encourage patients to walk while in the hospital. Many patients benefit from a visit from a physical therapist (PT) or occupational therapist (OT) while in the hospital. If you have any concerns about mobility, don't be afraid to ask for PT or OT referrals!

BEFORE LEAVING THE HOSPITAL

The patient, family, friends, and other loved ones need to know how to handle any drains, dressings, or other medical restrictions a patient has after surgery. I've found that drains are the most surprising to patients and families.

When we remove a mass or we mess with a body cavity in the operating room, the body will respond. The body responds by filling that newly created space with fluid. This fluid is often called a *seroma*. We want to drain that fluid out for a variety of reasons. Removing the fluid prevents pain and decreases the risk of infection. Drains placed in a cavity help prevent that fluid from building up. Many patients go home with drains in place. Everyone helping to take care of the patient should know how to take care of the drains.

Other practical information the patient's home-care team should ask the doctor include finding out what type of diet is allowed and when the patient can shower.

The family and friends need to feel like they have the tools to help take care of the patient at home. If patients and loved ones feel ill-equipped, it may be good to touch base with a social worker. Social workers can help locate resources for the patient, such as a visiting nurse. They may also help find transportation back and forth to doctor's appointments.

WHERE ARE THE RESULTS?

Just as with the biopsy, there can be some delay between the surgery and the final pathology report. This usually takes anywhere from five to seven days.

As mentioned before, the pathologist will look under the microscope at the tumor, tissue, and lymph nodes removed during surgery. The pathologist will also stain the tumor to help identify it, grade it, and in some cases send it for genetic analysis.

The surgeon will likely want to see the patient again two to three weeks after surgery. The surgeon can then assess the wound(s) and the patient's progress. Sometimes surgeons want to wait until that first appointment to discuss the pathology results; other times, they'll discuss results over the phone.

UNDER THE MICROSCOPE: SEEING IS BELIEVING

Staging revolves around the TNM system (see chapter 3 for details). Before surgery, doctors use clinical formation (exam and scans) to determine the *clinical stage* of the cancer. After a patient has gone through surgery, we repeat this process to ascertain the *pathological stage*.

The pathological stage may be completely different from the clinical stage. Why? Remember, our scans and clinical information aren't perfect. But in cancer, seeing is believing. That means that we trust what we see under a microscope more than we trust scans. The pathological staging from surgery (which is just a new *TNM* and *stage*) takes precedence over the clinical stage.

PATHOLOGICAL STAGING

The pathological staging determines the next treatment steps. It also informs patients and the teams involved about the risk of cancer spread. The pathology report often summarizes the TNM and includes staging and the diagnosis. It holds much of the key information about a patient's cancer.

I always suggest that patients ask for a copy of their pathology report. The pathology report and the information from scans constitute the most essential information about a patient's cancer. This brings us to the next common mistake I see patients make:

Mistake #6: Not asking for a copy of their pathology report after surgery or scan results

THE NEXT TREATMENT STEPS

The surgeon will review the pathology report and scans with the patient and family. The surgeon will then make the proper referrals to medical oncologists (who deliver chemotherapy and immunotherapy), radiation oncologists (who deliver radiation), and palliative care doctors (who help manage cancer symptoms). We'll discuss these doctors and their treatments more in the upcoming chapters.

Chapter Seven

Chemotherapy

Chemotherapy involves the use of drugs to treat cancer. Surprisingly, we can often kill cancer with enough chemotherapy. The trick is trying to limit toxicity to the patient while using chemotherapy.

If a surgeon is a gardener removing cancerous weeds by the roots, then chemotherapy is an herbicide used to further decrease the chances that the cancer—the weed—will come back.

For treatment, we need to exploit what makes cancer different from the normal cells of the body. Cancer is concerned about only one thing: dividing. Taking advantage of this difference is what allows chemotherapy and radiation to work.

There are many kinds of chemotherapy that work on cancer cells, but we can split them into two main types. The first is the classic drug that damages the DNA of the cancer cell. The second blocks the growth messages that are translated to the cell's proteins. Both look to damage or hinder the fundamental properties of a cancer cell.

CLASSIC CHEMOTHERAPY: ATTACKING DNA

Chemotherapy that damages the DNA of cancer cells also damages normal cells in the same way. The normal cells care deeply about that damage. They stop what they're doing, repair the damage, and then get back to their normal lives.

But cancer cells don't care about the damage; they're only concerned with trying to grow and divide. Damage from the chemotherapy continues to accumulate. When a cancer cell tries to divide, it has to make a copy of its DNA to pass on to the new cells. The DNA doesn't replicate properly because the cancer cell hasn't repaired the damage from chemotherapy. The cancer cell dies trying to pass on damaged DNA. In this way, chemotherapy targets cells that are dividing often (also known as fast-growing cells).

Normal cells that grow quickly are the ones most likely affected by chemotherapy. This includes cells of the gastrointestinal tract (gut, mouth, swallowing tube), hair, nails, and bone marrow (which makes blood cells). This explains many of the common side effects of chemotherapy: nausea, sores in the mouth, loss of hair or fingernails, and low blood counts.

Of course, different chemotherapies have different side effects. But this explanation gives you a basic understanding of how chemotherapy works and why side effects happen.

CHEMOTHERAPY THAT TARGETS CANCER CELLS

The second type of chemotherapy includes a wide range of drugs (molecules) that affect cell growth. Remember, a cell's DNA transcribes orders to the RNA, which builds proteins.

The proteins are the ones that do the heavy lifting; they do the tasks in or around the cells. These proteins can be found inside the cell or on the surface (the surface proteins are called *cell receptors*).

If chemicals are available to block the function of specific proteins, we can stop the cancer cell from growing or functioning. This therapy is more targeted. We're looking to stop a specific protein from working. Because this therapy is specific, it may have fewer side effects. This is how targeted chemotherapy works.

A pathologist may stain the tumor for certain proteins and perform genetic tests (see chapter 3). We can use that information on a patient's tumor to decide how to give targeted therapy.

Classic examples of targeted therapy come from inhibiting sex hormones in breast or prostate cancers. The protein receptors on certain cancer cells depend on the body's normal female or male hormones to function. Usually the hormones bind to the protein (receptor) and encourage the cancer cell to grow. One way we can interfere with this process is to block the hormones so they can't bind to the receptor. (This is how the medicine *tamoxifen* works in treating breast cancer.)

Or we can decrease the amount of hormones in the body so there are fewer hormones to connect to these proteins. The hormones are like gasoline for a fire. They turn on the proteins and urge the cell to grow or divide. If we remove the fuel, the fire dies down. This is the basis of androgen-deprivation therapy in treating prostate cancer. (A commonly used drug is *leuprolide*.)

There are now new forms of targeted chemotherapy that are even more specific. These new drugs target and bind proteins specific to cancer cells. By binding a specific protein, they inhibit the proteins' actions. This often stops the cancer cell from growing or dividing.

These targeted medications have a range of side effects. The side effects depend on what their targets are!

TARGETED THERAPY: THE ACHILLES' HEEL . . . FOR SOME

Reading about targeted therapy, it may sound like a real good solution to cancer. *Cancer cells have specific receptors, and we have drugs to target those receptors; that should lead to cures.* This approach to cancer treatment brought much enthusiasm in the 1990s and early 2000s. In fact, it did significantly change the landscape in some cancers. For example, *CML*, or chronic myelogenous leukemia, is a liquid tumor of the blood that used to have a high mortality rate. Back in the 1970s (before targeted therapy) less than 10% of CML patients survived ten years. However, a new drug was developed (*Gleevec*; see the glossary) that targets a certain mutation in this cancer. Now the long-term survival rate for patients with CML is greater than 90%!

So what's the problem?

Although targeted therapy works long-term for some cancers, for the majority of cancers, resistance to treatment develops over time. For example, in lung cancer, there is a particular mutation in a protein/ receptor called *EGFR* (see glossary). This receptor may be targeted by certain drugs, such as *Osimertinib* (see glossary). This mutation can lead to the development of lung cancer in young patients who were never smokers. In fact, the author of *When Breath Becomes Air* (highly recommended—please see the resources), Dr. Paul Kalanithi, was a young neurosurgeon who developed lung cancer with this mutation. His book describes his cancer journey in detail and is an eye-opening read for patients, loved ones, or anyone touched by cancer. He was given a targeted therapy, but eventually his cancer progressed over time.

The reason many of these cancers continue to grow after targeted therapy is that the drugs are not 100% effective. For example, in a one-centimeter cancer mass alone there are likely about one hundred million cells. If a targeted therapy was 99.9% effective, that would still leave one hundred thousand cancer cells alive and growing. These cells left behind are "resistant" to the treatment (hence why they survived the treatment). Those surviving cells may also be more aggressive in growing and dividing. We are always trying to develop drugs (new targeted therapy) to destroy these "resistant" cells. Many have made the analogy that this pursuit is like whack-a-mole: we're always trying to catch up to where the new resistance will pop up. It can be difficult to keep up.

Targeted therapies may hold a cancer back for months to years, but for many, the cancer may continue to grow and spread after some time. The resistance to targeted treatment depends on the target and the type of cancer. If you are on targeted therapy, it is important to discuss with your physician how long the average patient is on this treatment before any resistance may develop.

MAKING TREATMENT LESS TOXIC

What makes cancer deadly is its ability to spread. The benefit of chemotherapy is that it goes *everywhere*, so it can help attack cancer wherever it may be. The downside of chemotherapy is that it goes *everywhere*.

This means the side effects of treatment may occur in many parts of the body. Chemotherapy may affect the heart, lungs, gut, skin, or any other part. To help lessen these side effects, chemotherapy is often given in cycles.

A cycle of treatment is often followed by a period of rest. Most chemotherapy cycles are days to weeks in length. Cycles make up a *chemotherapy course* of all the cycles put together. The number of cycles will vary by the number of drugs and the type of cancer.

Patients should get some of the following information from their doctors:

• What does a cycle consist of?

- How much rest time is there?
- How many cycles make up this course of chemotherapy?

Medical oncologists (who give the chemotherapy) are terrific at mapping out a schedule of when chemotherapy will be given.

Make sure to define the goal of treatment with the medical oncologist. Although chemotherapy is often given as a curative treatment, it can be palliative. Even if a patient cannot be cured, chemotherapy can slow down cancer and prevent the development of cancer symptoms.

OTHER DRUGS:
HITTING CANCER WITH A ONE-TWO PUNCH

Chemotherapy is often given in combination with many other drugs. These combinations of drugs have fancy acronyms: *EPOCH*, *R-CHOP*, *AC-T*. (I define some of these for you in the glossary.) Often, each one of these letters stands for a different chemotherapy drug. There are hundreds of these combinations.

If you hear an acronym you don't understand, make sure to ask! Also record the start and stop dates of chemotherapy. These chemotherapy combinations may consist of one to ten drugs. We often use a combination because doing so makes it harder for cancer cells to resist treatment.

RECEIVING CHEMOTHERAPY

Some chemotherapy is given as a pill. Other chemotherapy is given directly into a vein. This is called *intravenous*, or IV, chemotherapy.

To avoid having the patient get poked with a needle every day, a *port*—sometimes called a *mediport* or *port-a-cath*—is placed, which consists of a quarter-sized disk that fits just under the skin. That disk is connected to tubing that goes to the heart. Nurses and doctors can access the port to draw blood or give chemotherapy.

We implant a port under the skin in a same-day procedure. The patient can go home the same day. After chemotherapy is over, we withdraw the port in another outpatient procedure. Some patients don't need a port. You can discuss the need for a port with your medical team.

CHEMOTHERAPY AND THEN SURGERY? OR SURGERY BEFORE CHEMOTHERAPY?

The timing of chemotherapy—before or after a surgery—depends on the situation. Traditionally, chemotherapy or radiation was given after most surgical procedures; this is called *adjuvant therapy*. A more recent movement in medicine involves giving chemotherapy before surgery.

By giving chemotherapy before surgery, we can better predict whether a person's cancer will respond to treatment. We can see the mass shrink in real time. If a tumor responds to chemotherapy, we know it's more likely that any cancer cells that may have metastasized (traveled to other parts of the body) will also respond to treatment.

Some cancers tend to spread to other parts of the body rapidly and early. In that scenario, giving chemotherapy before surgery makes sense, because it kills small amounts of that traveling disease.

Chemotherapy is also given before surgery to shrink the tumor. Shrinking the mass with chemotherapy may make it easier for the surgeon to completely remove the cancer. To remove all the microscopic disease, the surgeon won't have to remove as much normal tissue. Using chemotherapy or radiation before surgery is called *neoadjuvant therapy*. (This is also known as *induction therapy*.)

Patients can discuss the pros and cons of doing chemotherapy before or after surgery with their doctors.

For some tumors, shrinking the cancer before surgery isn't practical, and some tumors don't respond well to chemotherapy. Doctors and the medical team will tailor cancer treatment for each patient.

COMBINING CHEMOTHERAPY WITH RADIATION: THE LAWNMOWER APPROACH

Instead of giving chemotherapy as a mix of many drugs, single-agent (one-drug) chemotherapy is often given with radiation. Again, this can be given before or after surgery. (Examples of drugs commonly used with radiation are *cisplatin* and *capecitabine*. I describe some of these drugs in the glossary.)

Why would we give radiation with chemotherapy? They both damage the cancer cells, but they do so in slightly different ways (see the next chapter for info on radiation therapy). These types of chemotherapy drugs make a cancer cell more sensitive to the effects of radiation.

I often tell patients to picture a cancer cell as a weed lying flat on the lawn. A lawnmower, which in this case is the radiation, comes by to clip the plant. The lawnmower has a much harder job if the plant is lying flat. Chemotherapy forces the weed (the cancer cell) to stand tall so the lawnmower (the radiation) can cut it.

In the same way, chemotherapy gets the cancer cell ready for radiation's attack. In this scenario, the chemotherapy is sensitizing the cancer—making it more responsive—to radiation while also attacking cancer at the roots. The combination of chemotherapy with radiation is often known as *chemoradiation.*

So why use just one chemotherapy drug with radiation? Why not multiple drugs? Because in general, using many drugs is too toxic to the patient. Remember, we always try to balance the benefits of cancer treatment versus the likely side effects.

KNOW YOUR DRUGS: MEDICATION INTERACTION

Some supplements, over-the-counter medications, and prescription medications may interact with chemotherapy and even radiation! It's critical that the medical care team know exactly what medications a patient is taking.

Keep an up-to-date list of medications and supplements in a treatment binder (or other system you use to organize information). If you don't have such a list, put all the medications, supplements, and herbs a patient is taking in a clear plastic bag and bring them to the doctor's office. This will allow the team time to go through everything the patient is taking.

This is the next common mistake patients make:

Mistake #7: Not having an up-to-date list of medications and supplements for the doctors

DEALING WITH THE PRACTICAL ASPECTS
OF CHEMOTHERAPY

Chemotherapy is often given over many weeks to months. Patients and families should have a plan to help with the practical aspects of chemotherapy. This includes transportation (most often car rides) and managing things around the house. This is to help alleviate the mental and physical burden for the person undergoing cancer treatment.

Social workers are experts in helping patients work through the practical aspects of cancer care and also make up an important part of the emotional care team (see chapter 4).

I recommend that every patient meet with a social worker—even patients who think they already have everything they need. Patients are often surprised what social workers can help with. Unfortunately, many patients and families don't ask to meet with a social worker until there's a problem.

MONTHS OF TREATMENT . . . OR YEARS?

Targeted chemotherapy is often administered over long periods of time. These targeted therapies may be a pill taken daily or a shot given once every few months. These treatments may continue for weeks to years.

This also means experiencing some side effects over a long period. But in most scenarios, these types of targeted treatments are well tolerated and the side effects are manageable. Patients should speak to their doctor and make sure to record how long they'll be on any targeted therapies (weeks, months, or years).

CHEMOTHERAPY AND SIDE EFFECTS TO CONSIDER

The side effects of chemotherapy often depend on how the drugs work on fast-growing cells in the body. Some side effects occur during or shortly after treatment (*acute side effects*). Other side effects occur later. These are known as *late side effects* and they may appear months to years after treatment.

Acute side effects of treatment include fatigue, nausea, vomiting, taste changes, smell changes, diarrhea, constipation, hair loss, low blood counts (which increase risk of infection), mouth ulcers, liver dysfunction, and skin changes, among others.

Long-term effects of chemotherapy may include heart failure, nerve and sensation changes, scarring of the lung, fertility issues, and second cancers. Now, all this sounds scary, but not all patients will develop these side effects. Side effects depend on both the chemotherapy drugs used and the size of the dose a patient has received. For example, the risk of heart failure with a chemotherapy drug called *doxorubicin* directly depends on how big the dose is.

Common side effects of chemotherapy include low appetite and fatigue. I address these in depth later in the book, as we have specific ways to help cope with these changes (see chapter 12).

Maintaining weight is vital during chemotherapy (remember performance status?). Keeping up a patient's weight can help make sure they can fight off infection, heal properly, and get through treatment. This sometimes means getting nutrition through a feeding tube. I outline my thoughts on diet and feeding tubes in chapter 12.

By now I hope you realize that chemotherapy often affects fast-growing cells. This includes eggs and sperm, which may affect fertility. I urge patients to talk to their doctors early regarding family planning. If you want to do sperm or egg banking, try to do it before starting treatment. We'll discuss fertility and sexuality in chapter 12.

EVERYONE IS UNIQUE

Everyone responds to chemotherapy differently and will experience side effects uniquely. Even if your neighbor had the same cancer and treatment, don't assume they've had the same experience! Stay as organized as you can to help coordinate treatments.

Chapter Eight

Radiation Therapy

Many patients have a lot of fear and misconceptions about radiation treatment. Radiation is used to treat over 50% of patients with cancer. It's an important part of treatment. I outline how radiation works and its role in cancer treatment in this chapter.

HOW DOES RADIATION WORK?

Radiation treatment uses high-power X-rays to treat cancer. *X-rays* are electromagnetic waves (like light) but are in a spectrum that isn't visible to the human eye. We do have cameras that can see X-rays.

In a lot of ways, radiation works like chemotherapy. We try to use the differences between cancer cells and normal cells to our advantage.

High-power X-rays damage cells by making free radicals, called *oxidants*. The oxidants damage the DNA of both normal cells and cancer cells. Normal cells recognize the damage from the X-rays. They then halt what they're doing to repair the damage before they continue to grow or divide.

The cancer cells ignore the damage and keep trying to divide. This damage accumulates over time. Eventually the damage to the DNA is so great that the cell dies when it tries to copy its DNA. This is the rationale behind how radiation works. (Does this sound similar to chemotherapy that targets DNA? If it does, then good! It's a very similar process.)

You've likely heard of *anti*oxidants being good, so why would we want to make *oxidants*? The idea of *antioxidants* is that they prevent free-radical damage to the DNA of normal cells. Less damage means fewer mutations and a potentially lower risk for cancer over the long term. But once a patient has cancer, we want to make oxidants to treat cancer. Antioxidants given during cancer treatment could work to our disadvantage.

RADIATION: THE INVISIBLE SCALPEL

With radiation, we treat cancer without making an incision. We can destroy cancer cells in a certain part of the body while avoiding normal tissues. Radiation works locally, only at the spot we aim our X-rays.

Just as with surgery, there are side effects of radiation treatment. During treatment, the patient will meet with the radiation oncologist once a week to help manage the side effects.

The side effects of radiation therapy depend on where we aim the X-rays. This corresponds to where a doctor is cutting with their scalpel. If radiation is used to treat a tumor in the belly, a patient may experience nausea. If a patient is receiving radiation to the skin, that area will likely lose hair and may become red or irritated.

The effects of radiation are local. This differs from chemotherapy, which goes everywhere and so has systemic side effects. For example, if you give radiation to someone's feet, you wouldn't expect that person to lose the hair on their head.

DECISIONS, DECISIONS: TIMING AND FRACTIONS

The dose and timing of radiation treatment depends on the stage, location, and type of cancer. Many tumors respond to radiation differently. Some cancers are sensitive to it, and others are resistant. Doctors may choose to vary the dose of radiation given each day, depending on the goals of care (cure or pain control). A radiation oncologist, as part of the cancer team, helps decide whether to use radiation and how it should be incorporated into the treatment plan.

Tumors receive radiation treatment broken up into fractions, most often given every day or every other day, Monday through Friday. A *fraction* just refers to a single radiation treatment.

Breaking up the treatment into fractions allows cancer cells time to accumulate damage from radiation. It also gives normal cells time to repair damage.

Radiation may be given for a day, a week, or several weeks. The dose is measured in a unit called a *gray*. (See the glossary for a full definition.) This term is used to define the amount of energy we put into a tumor to try to destroy it.

MORE DISCUSSIONS AROUND SURGERY

Radiation therapy may be given before or after surgery. Before surgery, we can use it to shrink a tumor. This makes surgery easier by increasing the chances we'll get a *negative margin*—an area of disease-free tissue around the tumor.

But for some tumors, shrinking the cancer with radiation before surgery is impractical. In other cases, tumors don't respond well to radiation and won't shrink with treatment.

Most commonly, radiation is given after surgery. This may help decrease the chances the cancer will come back locally, in the same spot.

If surgery removes the cancer, why do we need radiation? As we pointed out before, cancer is like a weed stretching out its roots into normal tissue. No matter how good surgeons are, they can't see cells without a microscope in the operating room. That's why surgeons try to take an amount of normal-appearing tissue around the tumor during surgery.

It's always possible that some cancer cells will be left behind. If they're allowed to grow, they'll form a new mass. Radiation destroys these leftover cells to prevent the cancer from coming back.

RADIATION WITH CHEMO: LOWERING CANCER RISK, BOTH LOCAL AND SYSTEMIC

As a rule of thumb, radiation decreases the risk that cancer will come back after surgery by about half. This number varies significantly based on the type of cancer and location, but it's a good estimate.

This reduction applies only to the risk of local recurrence. Radiation doesn't lower the risk the cancer will come back somewhere else in the body. Remember, radiation works like a scalpel—the treatment is focused.

This is very different from chemotherapy, which goes everywhere. Chemotherapy lowers the risk cancer will come back in another part of the body. It destroys any of the cells that may have metastasized (moved to another area of the body).

Let's consider an example. Suppose Leslie's breast cancer is removed with surgery. Her pathology indicates that the risk of her cancer coming back at five years may be as high as 30%. By giving Leslie radiation, we lower the risk of her cancer coming back in the breast to 15% (half of the original risk). Notice that adding radiation doesn't make the risk 0%! But it does cut the risk in half: 15/30 = 1/2. A single cell left behind may be enough for a cancer to return.

Leslie may also benefit from hormonal therapy, as some cells may have escaped to other parts of her body that didn't respond to chemotherapy. Radiation will not address those cells, but chemotherapy will.

RADIATION AS PAIN CONTROL: A POWERFUL TOOL

Besides working to prevent the recurrence of cancer, radiation can also decrease pain from cancer. It's common for many cancers (breast, prostate, and others) to spread to bone. The cancer pushes on the normal bone, causing pain, discomfort, and even broken bones. Radiation directed at cancer in the bone helps destroy the cancer in that region and reduce pain. This is a common use for radiation in the palliative setting (noncurative treatment). About 60 to 70% of patients get pain relief from radiation in this way.

Radiation is also helpful to treat pain from cancer in other parts of the body, such as the liver, bowels, or brain.

TYPES OF RADIATION: AN ELECTRON, A PROTON, AND A PHOTON ALL ENTER A ROOM . . .

The treatment team will decide what type of radiation to use to treat a patient's cancer. Beyond the classic X-ray treatments we discussed earlier (an X-ray is a type of *photon*), we can use other types of radiation. The types of radiation treatment available are generally made from the parts of an atom.

Electrons are small negatively charged particles that we can use to treat skin or surface cancers. They don't penetrate far because they're so small.

Protons are large, positively charged particles used to treat cancer. They're becoming more popular because of some theoretical benefits over X-ray (photon) treatment. In most scenarios, clinical data isn't available to show that protons are better than X-ray radiation. Patients and doctors should talk at their appointments about the type of radiation that will be used.

RADIATION MACHINES AND TECHNIQUES

External radiation treatments may be given in a variety of ways by many types of machines. Some terms you may hear in the clinic include *IMRT (intensity-modulated radiation therapy)*, *TomoTherapy*, *Truebeam*, *VMAT (volumetric modulated arc therapy)*, *Gamma Knife*, *MRI-Guided*, and *Cyberknife*.

These fancy techniques and machines are used to give X-ray (photon) radiation. If you want to know the details, there's ample reading material out there. I've included descriptions for each term in the glossary as well.

Each machine and technique has its pros and cons. No machine has a special advantage over another. Don't base your decision to pursue treatment on special advertising of a certain machine.

GETTING READY FOR RADIATION

Once a patient and doctor agree that radiation should be part of the treatment plan, the patient goes through a CT (CAT) simulation scan. This CT scan is just like a diagnostic CT scan (see chapter 3), except this scan is used to plan the radiation.

For the scan, the patient will be set up in the treatment position. This position depends on the site of the body being treated. Often a mold is made to fit around the patient and keep them in the same place each day. For cancers of the head, neck, and throat, we make each patient a customized mask out of a thin plastic material.

Accuracy in setup is essential. The goal of radiation is to treat the cancer while sparing as much normal tissue as possible. We want to make sure the patient is in the correct position each day of treatment. If a patient is in the wrong place, we could miss the tumor or hit normal structures. We often make three marks on patients. We use these marks to line up patients to lasers in the CT simulation and treatment room. That helps us know a patient is in the right position.

After a CT simulation scan, the radiation oncologist works with a team to design a patient's radiation. (Notice a pattern? Everything in cancer treatment needs a team!) A doctor works with a *dosimetrist* (someone specializing in how to calculate radiation doses) and a *medical physicist* (someone with a master's degree or PhD in physics) to come up with a patient's unique radiation plan.

WHAT TO EXPECT DURING RADIATION TREATMENT

Treatment appointments last from 15 to 45 minutes, but this can vary with the type of treatment.

Radiation therapists help cancer patients get set up on the treatment table at the treatment machine. The machine we use to deliver the radiation is called a *linear accelerator.* (This is a generic name. Many companies make different types of linear accelerators. I mentioned a few earlier: TomoTherapy, Truebeam, etc.)

Once the patient is on the treatment table, an image is often taken to confirm that the patient is in the right place. Then the treatment is given, lasting from 2 to 20 minutes. Often, more time is spent setting a patient up on the treatment table than doing the treatment. A patient doesn't feel anything during radiation treatment; it's like getting a chest X-ray.

After each external radiation treatment, a patient is *not* radioactive. Patients should feel free to engage with loved ones, children, and animals.

GETTING TO AND FROM APPOINTMENTS: TRANSPORT FOR RADIATION TREATMENTS

Making daily trips back and forth to the hospital for radiation treatments can be challenging. Patients who live far from the radiation center may ask their doctors if there's a radiation oncology clinic closer to home. Often there isn't. Radiation machines cost millions of dollars, and not every hospital has them available. Patients can connect with social workers to help with car rides, bus services, or housing to get to treatment.

BRACHYTHERAPY: INTERNAL RADIATION

There's a type of treatment where we implant radiation directly in the tumor. This is called *brachytherapy*.

Sometimes this involves leaving radioactive material in the body. For example, prostate seed implants are a type of brachytherapy. Doctors place the seeds, a type of radioactive material, in the prostate. The seeds give off X-rays that travel only a short distance, killing cancer cells but sparing nearby normal organs. The radiation is given off slowly as the material decays. When the material has decayed, it no longer gives off X-rays.

Some brachytherapy treatments do not leave a radioactive source inside a person. Instead, a localized radiation treatment is given via a radioactive source, and then the source is removed. This sometimes requires multiple trips for treatment. This approach is a common way to treat cervical or uterine cancer.

Why would we bother to do this when we have external radiation? Brachytherapy is much more localized, so there may be fewer side effects to nearby normal organs. In the case of the prostate, there could be less irritation of the nearby bladder or rectum (bowel). For many patients, we combine external beam radiation and brachytherapy to maximize the dose to tumors.

Some internal radiation treatments can make patients radioactive for a period of time. If you have any questions about being around children or animals after treatment, ask the radiation oncologist.

IMMEDIATE AND LATE SIDE EFFECTS OF RADIATION

We break up side effects of radiation into two types: immediate and late.

Immediate side effects (*acute side effects*) take place during radiation or within a month after treatment. The acute side effects of radiation peak one to two weeks after treatments are finished.

Why would the side effects peak after radiation is done? Well, remember, normal cells see the damage to the DNA and stop what they're doing. They then take time to process and repair that damage.

This takes time, as damage has accumulated over the course of a radiation treatment. Therefore, while this repair is ongoing in normal tissues, the side effects are slightly delayed.

The acute side effects of radiation treatment may include skin redness, dry skin, sore throat, problems swallowing, fatigue, low appetite, nausea, vomiting, diarrhea, and painful urination. This depends on the part of the body being treated by radiation.

In the long term (months to years after treatment), radiation can also cause damage to other organs. Examples of *late side effects* include heart issues, lung scarring, skin darkening or thickening, dry mouth, trouble swallowing, and arm or leg swelling.

I would stress that side effects depend on where in the body the radiation is targeted. Just like everyone reacts to chemotherapy differently, everyone reacts to radiation differently. The response is individual, just like cancers are individual.

RADIATION AND NEW CANCER RISK

Radiation does pose a risk of causing another cancer. This is called a *secondary cancer*. That idea is scary for many patients.

With modern radiation techniques, this risk is very low: a 1 to 2% risk of a cancer within the next 20 years after treatment. The risk varies across the type of cancer, the area treated, and the age of the patient. Patients can discuss this risk with their doctors.

THE THREE ORIGINAL PILLARS: SURGERY, CHEMOTHERAPY, AND RADIATION

In closing, radiation is a pillar in the treatment of cancer. It can work with surgery to lower the risk of local recurrence or be used as a standalone treatment. It can also be helpful for pain control. Patients should ask doctors on their medical team whether radiation should be part of the treatment plan.

Surgery, chemotherapy, and radiation are the three original pillars of cancer treatment. In the next chapter, we'll discuss the newest pillar: immunotherapy.

Chapter Nine

The Future of Cancer Care

Immunotherapy, the Gray Zone, and Clinical Trials

This chapter will review the newest landscape in cancer care. This includes immunotherapy, curing patients with radiation and surgery like never before, and clinical trials pushing our knowledge forward.

Immunotherapy is now the fourth pillar in treating cancer, along with surgery, radiation, and chemotherapy. Being able to harness the power of the immune system to fight cancer has been a dream of cancer doctors for generations.

As seen in chapter 2, one of the hallmarks of cancer is its skill at evading the immune system. If cancer is a criminal and the immune system is the cops chasing it, then cancer cells are constantly throwing up smoke screens. They're trying to confuse, outrun, and hide from the immune system. The cancer can even cause the immune system to turn against itself. Cancer cells can confuse the immune system and cause it to shut down at the wrong times!

New drugs turn the immune system on to recognize cancer cells. Years of work have gone into making these drugs. At the cellular level, these drugs basically get rid of any traitors in the immune system. Cancer cells are hiding behind smoke and mirrors. These drugs allow the immune system to see through the cancer cells' disguise and hunt them down.

NOT MAGIC BUT GETTING CLOSE

Immunotherapy drugs are relatively new, so we don't know their effects across many different types of cancers. There's lots of data that these drugs help treat lung cancer, melanoma, renal cell carcinoma, head and neck cancers, and many other types of cancers (see the glossary for different immunotherapy drugs, including *durvalumab, nivolumab*, and *pembrolizumab*). This field is rapidly expanding and evolving, and new indications for immunotherapy seem to come out every month. For example, immunotherapy is now part of the standard treatment of advanced lung cancer. These drugs have had a major impact on how cancer is controlled and how long patients are living. Of patients with metastatic lung cancer (Stage IV patients), less than 5% (1 in 20 patients) used to make it to five years. With these new immunotherapies, we are now seeing 20% (one in five) of patients alive at five years! Although these numbers are still less than ideal, they represent a huge improvement.

The effectiveness of immunotherapy is being studied across many cancers in the United States. Taking part in a clinical trial may allow a patient access to these medicines (more on this later in the chapter). Different types of immunotherapy drugs have distinct effectiveness across various cancers. In fact, combining some different immunotherapies may lead to better outcomes. But this comes at the cost of more side effects.

There's a lot of potential for these drugs in the clinic. Unfortunately for most patients, these drugs are not a cure for advanced disease (Stage IV cancers). They stand as another pillar working with surgery, radiation, and chemotherapy to treat cancer. However, we do see a small number of patients who have long-term survival with these new drugs.

TUMOR TESTING: WILL I BENEFIT FROM IMMUNOTHERAPY?

Not every patient will benefit from immunotherapy. Doctors and scientists are still trying to determine which patients are most responsive to immunotherapies (and what types of immunotherapy to use for each different cancer). A biopsy or a tumor removed from a patient may be "tested" for certain changes that make it more responsive to certain immunotherapy, chemotherapy, or targeted treatments. It may be important to ask your medical team if the tumor sample was tested for certain markers such as *PD-1/PD-L1* or *TMB* (see glossary for scientific definitions). This may help predict if a patient would benefit from immunotherapy. Many of these tests have become standard across different cancer types, but it is often worth asking your doctor if you or your loved one's tumor or biopsy was tested.

At this time, we do not completely understand immunotherapy. Some patients still benefit from immunotherapy even without the markers I mentioned. Patients, family members, and loved ones should discuss with the medical treatment team the potential benefits of immunotherapy in the context of their cancer.

SIDE EFFECTS OF AN OVERLY ACTIVE IMMUNE SYSTEM

Most of these immunotherapies work by releasing the brake on the immune system. The idea is that if we turn on the immune system, cancer cells can no longer hide themselves. But this is a nonspecific activation of the immune system: the immune system is overly active everywhere, throughout the body. This gives us clues about many of the potential side effects of these drugs.

There's a huge presence of the immune cells in the skin, gut, and lungs, but these cells are not often very active. These immunotherapy drugs turn on the immune system where it's normally quiet. Therefore, side effects can be significant.

These side effects may include skin redness, nausea, vomiting, liver damage, diarrhea, lung damage, or cough. Immunotherapy medications may also lead to abnormal hormone levels (the immune system reacts against normal glands) or even death (from an immune reaction leading to multiple organs failing). These drugs hold significant promise, but make no mistake—they can have serious side effects!

RADIATION IMPROVING IMMUNOTHERAPY: SOMETIMES LUCK HAS A LOT TO DO WITH IT

Doctors noticed an interesting trend in the early days of radiation treatment. Once in a while, they would treat a tumor in one part of the body with radiation (for example the hip). As that tumor shrank in response, a tumor in another area of the body (for example, the lung) would sometimes began to shrink too, even though the tumor in the lung had never been targeted by the radiation. This happened rarely but was seen multiple times over decades of treatment. Didn't I say radiation worked like a scalpel? It only works where you aim the radiation? Then what was happening here?

We didn't understand why this happened until recently. Researchers found that destroying a tumor in one part of the body with radiation helps the immune system recognize cancer cells in another part of the body. This idea is known as the *abscopal effect*.

Although interesting, the abscopal effect was erratic and only an interesting scientific observation. However, with new immunotherapy treatments, we find that radiation and immunotherapy can work better together: The radiation helps the body "see" the cancer (that had been hiding from the immune system), and the immunotherapy "turns on" the immune system to attack it. Combining radiation to one area of the body with immunotherapy may lead to better responses to treatment throughout the body. We are studying this effect more in clinical trials.

IMMUNOTHERAPY MAY IMPROVE CHEMOTHERAPY

Immunotherapy is also changing the way chemotherapy is used across cancers. In some cancers, we have found that immunotherapy works better than chemotherapy. For other cancers, combining chemotherapy with immunotherapy leads to better outcomes. Chemotherapy destroys cancer cells as described in previous chapters, and the immunotherapy turns on the immune system to attack cancer cells that survive. However, the more treatments given together, the higher the toxicity. Therefore a balance must be struck between treatments administered and side effects.

THE CHALLENGE AND FUTURE OF IMMUNOTHERAPY

There are other drawbacks to immunotherapy. Immunotherapy drugs are costly. In fact, some newer drugs cost more per gram than gold. Keep this in mind if out-of-pocket payment is a consideration. These drugs may be available through clinical trials. And recall that these drugs turn on the immune system in general; this can lead to major side effects for patients. Despite these obstacles, this new pillar of treatment holds significant promise.

Our goal is to turn on the immune system in specific ways to target cancer but not overstimulate the immune system everywhere in the body. This will be done by developing new drugs. Combining radiation or chemotherapy together with immunotherapy to help it work better is a promising approach. Other researchers are using vaccines (developed against cancer) to help the immune system better identify cancer cells. All these approaches will continue to work together to improve outcomes for patients.

This new therapy has given hope to many patients and family members.

LIMITED-DISTANT CANCER SPREAD AND TREATMENT: THE GRAY ZONE

In an earlier chapter (chapter 5), I emphasized that doctors need to spell out the goals of care for patients and family members. The two main options for treatment are curative or palliative intent. However, our understanding of cancer and how that affects goals of care are changing rapidly. This is because there exists a spectrum of cancer spread from when a cancer moves from curable to incurable. This "gray zone" makes determining the goals of care difficult. It makes it hard to know the right thing to do.

LIMITED-DISTANT SPREAD OF DISEASE: WHAT DOES IT IMPLY?

During the workup process, we described the TNM staging system (chapter 3), where tumor, lymph nodes, and metastasis are considered. As a reminder, a cancer *metastasizes* when it spreads to other organs (liver, lungs, and so on).

Once cancer has spread (or metastasized) to other organs, the cancer is considered to be advanced (usually Stage IV disease, depending on the cancer). In most instances, Stage IV cancer is considered to be incurable. Recently doctors have made some interesting observations that challenge this assumption for some patients. Those people with only a few sites of distant cancer spread to other organs (usually limited to between one and five sites, depending on the type of cancer) have different outcomes than patients who may have disease spread all over the body.

Those people with limited spread of their cancer tend to have better outcomes than other people with multiple organs of involvement. This limited spread of disease to only a few sites is called *oligometastatic disease* (see glossary for a more detailed definition). Consider a patient who has a colorectal cancer that has spread to the liver as the only site of metastasis—that is, it's the only *distant disease spread* (please see glossary). Many of these patients undergo removal of part of the liver (even though the cancer has spread through the body to get to the liver). As long as the liver is the only site of disease, a number of these patients will be "cured" with surgery and chemotherapy. However, it is important to emphasize that only a small subset of these patients may be "cured" by this aggressive approach.

CAN WE REGROW THE GARDEN?

Let's go back to our garden analogy. If the entire garden is taken over by weeds (cancer), it is unlikely we are going to be able to remove all the weeds and save the garden. However, if there are only one to five weeds spread across the garden, we may be able to remove the weeds and save the rest of the normal plants of the garden (our normal body and organs).

For those of you who garden, there is an unfortunate truth in gardening that if you have a few weeds, you will likely have many, many more you can't see. These weeds may be hidden under the soil, where seeds are beginning to take hold. This is why new weeds are constantly popping up even if we remove the weeds we can see. Our bodies are very similar. The five cancer sites may be all the cancers the patient has. Or, alternatively, those five may be the only visible cancers, and many other sites of cancer are beginning to grow. We just can't see them yet.

A number of patients with limited disease spread still have an opportunity for cure. However, that is still a small number. As physicians, we do not know which patients with limited disease spread are curable. Because some patients within this limited disease spread are curable, it is tempting to treat everyone in this category with aggressive treatment. The problem is that lots of aggressive treatment comes with side effects, and we do not know who will benefit from this approach. In that context, patients, family members, loved ones, and everyone in this scenario needs to have an open and honest discussion with the medical team.

Do not forget mistake #3! Do not be afraid to ask questions. Some questions to consider concerning the aggressive treatment of patients with limited spread of their cancer (oligometastatic disease) include:

1. What is the best possible outcome with aggressive treatment? How likely is this outcome?
2. What is the worst possible outcome with aggressive treatment? How likely is this outcome?
3. Are there alternative treatments? Surgery? Radiation? Chemotherapy? Immunotherapy?
4. What would you consider standard of care?
5. Are there clinical trials available? (See the next few sections in this chapter for more on clinical trials.)

UNDERSTANDING LIMITED SPREAD THROUGH CLINICAL STUDIES

Doctors and researchers are only beginning to understand patients with limited disease spread (*oligometastatic disease*). We need to better understand who will benefit from aggressive therapy and who will not. It is important to understand the potential pros and cons of treatment in this setting.

Most importantly, there are many clinical trials that are looking to help clarify the right course of action for patients. I would encourage any patient in this scenario to enroll in a clinical trial. We will review clinical trials in the next section and the potential benefits of enrolling

WHAT IS A CLINICAL TRIAL?

In oncology, clinical trials are trying to answer a question about a drug, a treatment, or another intervention. The idea is to study a new treatment in people to better understand its effects and possibly improve outcomes.

THE PHASES OF A CLINICAL TRIAL

Clinical trials are broken up into phases 1 through 4. The goal of a clinical trial depends on which phase of study it's in.

- *Phase 1*: The safety of a drug or intervention is assessed. The goal is to determine the safe doses or side effects of a new treatment.
- *Phase 2*: A drug or treatment is given to a big group of people to see if it's effective and to further test out its safety.
- *Phase 3*: The drug or treatment is given to a large group (bigger than the phase 2 group) to confirm that it's better than or equal to standard treatments (or to a placebo if no standard is available).
- *Phase 4*: Long-term effects of the drug in the population are assessed.

Some clinical trials help a patient, but they may also help the next generation of patients.

WHY SHOULD I PARTICIPATE IN A CLINICAL TRIAL?

Clinical studies help keep medicine moving forward as we try to find better treatments for cancer and other diseases. We're in debt to every patient and family who has helped advance medicine by taking part in a clinical trial.

I urge patients to discuss clinical studies with their doctor. Participation in a clinical study may give patients access to the latest advances in modern medicine. An additional bonus is helping to improve outcomes for patients for generations to come.

If you want to look for ongoing clinical trials, I recommend visiting ClinicalTrials.gov for an up-to-date list. The American Cancer Society also has great information on current clinical trials at https://www.cancer.org/treatment/treatments-and-side-effects/clinicaltrials.html or call them at 1-800-303-5691 to speak with a specialist to help identify clinical trials that may benefit a particular patient.

Doctors are always looking for ways to move medicine forward both in and out of clinical trials. This includes incorporating complementary medicine into treatment, which we'll discuss in the next chapter.

BEYOND HELPING FUTURE SCIENCE

Some patients worry that participation in a clinical trial may lead to worse care. Multiple scientific studies have shown that patients receiving care in a clinical trial often receive superior care to what they might have otherwise received. Many experts consider clinical trial care the highest standard of cancer care. I encourage all patients and family members to consider participating in a clinical trial.

Chapter Ten

Integrative Medicine

Caring for the Whole Person

Many people think that Western medicine has brushed off all aspects of complementary and integrative therapy. Not true! The National Cancer Institute (NCI), the main center of funding for cancer research in the United States, has a whole branch dedicated to studying complementary treatments! We're always looking for new ways to treat cancer or manage side effects anywhere we can.

I do not advocate *alternative medicine*—using supplements or other nontraditional medications in place of traditional therapy—for cancer. A recent study from Yale shows that patients that pursue only alternative or complementary medicine without any standard cancer treatment have double the risk of death from cancer (https://www.ncbi.nlm.nih.gov/pubmed/30027204).

On the other hand, *complementary* therapies used along with traditional cancer treatment may provide significant benefits (although this is the most common definition of alternative and complementary medicines—some will alternate between these terms). The approach combining all aspects of care is known as *integrative medicine*.

In this chapter, I outline some complementary medicines and their integration with traditional care. Some of these therapies may have some benefits for patients; others may not. I also address some controversies around a few alternative medicine treatments.

I want to stress that these treatments should fit into the medical and emotional support teams' treatment plans. They're to work *with* standard treatments, not in place of them.

DOES *NATURAL* EQUAL *SAFE*?

Many patients understandably want to use natural products to fight cancer. Intuitively, we figure that nature will provide us with medications that may help combat disease. In many ways, this is true! Chemotherapies, antibiotics, and other medical advances often come from nature. For example, the bark of the Pacific yew tree, native to the Pacific Northwest of the United States, is used to derive paclitaxel, a common chemotherapy drug. *Paclitaxel* is used to treat breast or lung cancer.

Many patients then make the leap that *all* natural products are safe. This couldn't be further from the truth. Coming directly from nature doesn't mean that a product has cancer-fighting properties or is safe to use. Mercury and lead are both natural elements, but we know that ingesting mercury or lead can lead to significant poisoning.

Nature can help us against cancer. But we must use our knowledge to properly adapt cancer-fighting therapies from nature.

ACUPUNCTURE: GETTING POKED WITH NEEDLES

Acupuncture has a long history in Chinese medicine. It involves stimulating certain parts of the body by inserting needles. The idea of acupuncture is to balance the *qi* or life force of the body. Acupuncture may help some patients manage the side effects of cancer treatment.

Acupuncture is generally safe, especially when practiced by licensed and trained providers. There's some clinical evidence that acupuncture may help relieve nausea and vomiting (specifically those related to chemotherapy). Also, some studies show acupuncture may help relieve different kinds of pain.

Generally acupuncture can be integrated with standard cancer treatments. But it's important that doctors clear a patient before they undergo acupuncture.

BIOFIELD THERAPY: THE TRANSFER OF ENERGY

Biofield therapy includes a variety of practices: Healing Touch, therapeutic touch, and Reiki (from the Japanese tradition). These practices involve the energy transfer from the provider to the patient through a biofield, with limited physical contact.

Several studies have looked at whether these treatments help reduce anxiety and pain. There have been some positive results, but it's unclear whether this is due to chance. There's minimal to no risk with these therapies, as they involve no touching or physical intervention.

Used along with cancer treatment, biofield therapy may help patients deal with cancer and side effects. Many patients find the process relaxing. Biofield therapy can integrate with standard treatments with minimal risk.

MASSAGE THERAPY AND MUSIC THERAPY

Massage and music therapies may help lower stress, depression, and muscle tension and improve sleep. Limited clinical data is available on the efficacy of their use for cancer patients, but intuitively these therapies make sense for many.

Cancer can spread to bone, often in the spine. If the cancer has spread to bone, doctors should clear a patient before they get a massage. This is to make sure the bones in the back are stable enough to withstand significant pressure from a massage.

If a patient has worsening back pain with a known diagnosis of cancer, a doctor should evaluate this pain. This is to make sure the back pain isn't caused by cancer spreading to bone.

Music therapy needs no medical clearance. (I suggest '80s rock. Very relaxing!)

YOGA

Just like music therapy, biofield therapy, or acupuncture, yoga involves minimal risk. And like other forms of exercise, yoga may help improve mood, outlook, anxiety, depression, and other symptoms.

The key to integrating yoga is the same as for any exercise plan: Don't push exercise too hard or too fast. Mix it into life before, during, and after treatment to improve overall health.

SPINAL MANIPULATION

Spinal manipulation is a therapy that involves moving a spine joint to the end of its clinical range. (In a practical sense, this means bending it as far as it can go.) It's commonly used to treat back pain. I won't dive into all the controversies around spinal manipulation, but I will discuss spinal manipulation in the context of cancer.

I tell patients to be cautious about getting spinal manipulation after a cancer diagnosis for a few reasons. The first is that worsening back pain could indicate cancer is spreading to bones in the back. Spinal manipulation could hurt frail bones that are under attack by cancer. This could put a patient at a higher risk of breaking a bone with manipulation.

Before a patient undergoes any spinal manipulation, they should speak with a member of the medical team.

MARIJUANA

Patients often ask about marijuana as a part of their cancer treatment. Laws vary by state on the use of medical marijuana. Patients may want to check the laws of the state where they reside or receive treatment.

Many claims are made about the role of marijuana, from curing cancer to managing side effects. A big takeaway is that marijuana will not cure cancer, despite what many people may claim online. But marijuana may help improve mood, relieve nausea, and increase appetite, allowing some patients to eat and keep weight on.

Clinical studies have looked into the effectiveness of marijuana in helping patients with symptoms such as nausea. There's limited information comparing marijuana to better and more recently developed antinausea drugs. Regardless of the form of ingestion (by pill, oil, etc.), there's no good clinical evidence that marijuana has anticancer properties.

THC, the main psychoactive compound in marijuana, is made in pill form under the name *dronabinol*. This may be prescribed as a drug to improve appetite and decrease nausea. There are also other derivatives of marijuana, such as oils or solutions (sometimes called *cannabinoid oils* or *CBD oils*) that are focused on extracting the compound known as cannabidiol rather than the psychoactive THC.

CBD oils are becoming more popular as a remedy for cancer side effects and many other diseases. The evidence for their effectiveness is weak. The cost of CBD oil continues to go up. If you or a loved one use CBD oil, please inform your medical team. Do not spend large amounts of money on this treatment. CBD oil is largely unregulated, and the quality of what you are getting is unknown.

Downsides of marijuana use include elevated heart rate, poor judgment, sluggish motor skills, lung damage, and paranoia. Other concerns include the risk of infection (especially if smoked). Fungus spores residing in the plant when smoked could lead to lung infections, especially in people with low blood counts.

Patients should talk to their doctor to see if marijuana may help them.

HERBS AND SUPPLEMENTS

There are so many herbal supplements used to try to treat cancer and manage side effects that I could write a whole book on the subject. Some people have!

As mentioned earlier, people often assume that *natural* means *safe* or *effective*. Nature does provide us with some of our best cancer medicines and treatments! But many herbs and supplements can harm us.

Because supplements aren't strictly regulated, it's always unclear what you're getting in the bottle or pill. Some herbs and supplements may work against treatments such as chemotherapy or radiation.

Patients taking herbs or supplements should discuss them with their medical teams to make sure everyone is on the same page.

HIGH-DOSE VITAMIN C

I want to make special note of high-dose vitamin C, as this is a common alternative medicine treatment.

The idea behind high-dose vitamin C is that antioxidant effects can prevent cancer or prevent the progression of cancer. Vitamin C gets rid of free radicals that damage the body and DNA. However, there's little evidence that high doses of vitamin C prevent cancer.

Some clinical studies have assessed the benefits of high-dose vitamin C in treating advanced cancer. So far, vitamin C on it's own has failed to show any significant activity against tumors. There still are some studies trying to combine vitamin C with traditional cancer therapy.

Many alternative medicine providers will prescribe vitamin C and charge huge sums of money. Vitamin C is generally safe, as it's a water-soluble vitamin (the body excretes it through the urine, so it doesn't build up). But it may interact with certain chemotherapies.

Let your medical team know if this is something you're pursuing. I don't want to see patients pay high costs for care for no benefit. High-dose vitamin C shouldn't be used in place of traditional cancer therapies.

JUICING

If you Google "cancer juicing," you'll get hundreds of thousands of results. The idea is to extract juices from nutritious foods (fruits and vegetables) and use their antioxidant effects to prevent or treat cancer. Remember, oxidants damage the DNA of normal cells.

Taking in fruits and vegetables is a good thing. But some people claim you can fight cancer with juicing in place of surgery, chemotherapy, and radiation. There's no evidence to support this, and doing so may be dangerous.

I urge patients to keep a healthy and balanced diet. But do not replace standard cancer therapies with juicing.

"WHAT ARE YOU SELLING?": WATCHING OUT FOR SCAMS

There are so many alternative therapies available that I can't address them all here. The challenge for doctors and patients is that so much misinformation exists. So, whom should you trust when reading about cancer?

I understand why many people don't trust the medical establishment. At times we've rightfully lost that trust. But overall I think doctors, nurses, patient advocates, counselors, and others in the medical community are trying to do what we think is best for our patients. I watch colleagues work day and night, looking high and low to find new treatments for cancer.

Remember, cancer is not one disease but millions of diseases. Thus, we're looking for millions of individual cures for cancer. We all want a cure for this disease so badly. Unfortunately, this makes it easy for con artists to prey on our fears, anxiety, and hopes.

Always critically evaluate information. Ask yourself, "Is this person looking out for me, my friends, and my family, or are they just trying to profit off of me?"

Knowing whom to trust and what to believe in the realm of cancer can be hard. There are people out there looking to exploit patients and families through false hopes or flat-out lies. I don't want to see you, your friends, or your loved ones getting taken advantage of. As with all things in life, if something seems too good to be true, it probably is.

Chapter Eleven

Palliative Care and Hospice

Increasing Comfort

Treating cancer means taking care of the whole patient—the physical, the emotional, and the spiritual. This starts at diagnosis and carries through treatment and beyond.

Unfortunately, for some patients, cancer does find ways to spread that can cause physical pain, emotional strain, and difficulties in dealing with end-of-life issues. Palliative care and hospice providers are experts in helping people deal with these difficult times. These providers are an important part of the cancer care team.

WHAT IS PALLIATIVE CARE?

People are often petrified of the terms *palliative care* and *hospice*. Palliative care providers form part of a patient's care team. One of the biggest mistakes patients make is failing to get palliative care and hospice doctors involved in their care early on.

Palliative care provides specialized medical care to help relieve pain, stress, and symptoms from an illness. Palliative care providers can and should be part of the medical team! They work with patients with all types of significant medical challenges, such as heart failure, and play a key role in their care.

DEALING WITH PHYSICAL AND EMOTIONAL PAIN

Cancer and its treatment may cause pain or difficulty during normal activities. Medical oncologists, radiation oncologists, and surgeons are experts in dealing with pain and other side effects of cancer. Sometimes pain and other symptoms don't respond to our normal tricks or medications. That's where palliative care providers can help. They're clinicians with extra special training in dealing with these issues.

Emotional pain is often ignored in dealing with cancer (see chapter 4). Palliative care specialists receive training to help with the emotional aspects of grave illness, too. They work well with counselors, psychologists, social workers, and psychiatrists.

WHAT IS HOSPICE CARE?

Many palliative care providers also work in *hospice care*—or the end-of-life care that supports the patient, family, and loved ones as they face an advanced illness.

All medical care should emphasize quality of life, but hospice care takes this idea to the extreme. Active treatment is no longer given if it could artificially prolong suffering. The goal is for the patient to live well with minimal suffering.

Patients enter hospice when they likely have less than six months to live. The care can take place in a facility or at home.

There are many misconceptions about hospice care that I hope to clear up. Entering hospice doesn't mean that a patient will be stuck there! If a patient shows dramatic improvement, they can leave hospice care as well.

Active cancer treatment is generally not allowed while a patient is in hospice. Some hospice programs allow patients to receive radiation to decrease pain or other palliative treatments. Other hospice services need the patient to come off of hospice to get treated, and then patients reenroll in hospice. For most patients, this doesn't present a problem.

Entering hospice does not mean the care team is giving up on someone; rather, the care a patient can receive in hospice supports their journey of life and beyond. Just because a patient enters hospice doesn't mean that other providers don't want to be involved in their care. Doctors, nurses, and the medical and emotional support teams will follow along with the patient through hospice and end of life.

The transition to hospice is an emotional one. Both the medical and emotional support teams can help patients and families navigate this change.

EARLY INVOLVEMENT, BETTER OUTCOMES

Involving palliative care and hospice care doctors is not giving up on a person; it's just taking care of them as a whole.

Patients often wait to make palliative care treatment part of their cancer care. When things have gotten out of control—the pain is unbearable or they're struggling emotionally—then they ask for a palliative care consultation. There's no reason to wait!

Studies show that involving palliative care clinicians early improves outcomes for gravely ill patients. This includes improved survival, shorter hospital stays, fewer ER visits, and improvements in the quality of care.

Palliative care doctors often help with end-of-life issues, but that's only a fraction of what they do. They're incredible people who have a lot to offer. Don't be afraid to ask your medical team for a palliative care referral!

Similarly, the early involvement of hospice benefits patients. Studies show that when patients get hospice care involved early, they tend to live longer and have a better quality of life. Many patients and families don't get hospice care involved until late in treatment, often out of fear. It's the next common mistake that patients and families make.

Mistake #8: Waiting until very late into treatment or until the end of life to involve palliative care (pain management) or hospice care (end-of-life treatment). All cancer care needs to consider the whole patient.

In the next chapter, we'll delve into two more aspects of taking care of the whole person: nutrition and lifestyle.

Chapter Twelve

Lifestyle Changes to Improve Quality of Life and Outcomes

Nutrition and lifestyle are key to healthy living during and after cancer treatment. This chapter outlines the importance of managing diet, exercise, sexuality and fertility, and other areas of your life.

A HEALTHY DIET AND WEIGHT

There's no single food that's been found to prevent or cure cancer. Of course, you'll find many diet books and websites claiming otherwise. What we do know is that eating a healthy diet and exercising can lower the risk of many cancers, such as breast, colon, and endometrial cancer.

Keeping a healthy weight helps patients get through treatment. This will help patients stay as active as possible, heal, and fight off infections. A healthy diet is an essential part of developing a healthy body weight.

I suggest patients stick with the foods in a Mediterranean diet: plant-based foods (fruits, vegetables, nuts, and whole grains), fish, and poultry. This is a heart-healthy diet to adopt at any time in life. It involves replacing butter with olive oil and limiting red meat.

Foods to avoid include greasy, fatty, and fried foods, which are often associated with worse symptoms during cancer treatment. Many diets need adjustment to deal with nausea, diarrhea, cramping, changes in taste or smell, or trouble swallowing.

MAINTAINING WEIGHT

I want to stress the importance of keeping up a patient's weight during cancer treatment. Many studies of cancer patients have shown that those who lose a significant amount of weight have worse outcomes. The patients who lose weight have trouble getting through treatment. These patients have slow healing from surgery or develop other problems.

To keep weight on during cancer treatment, we aim for patients to take in 1,200 to 1,500 calories a day. I suggest that patients eat multiple small meals throughout the day rather than one to three huge meals. Eating many small meals allows a patient to get more calories without feeling sick from being full. As with most things in life, the slow and steady approach often wins out.

DRINK, DRINK, DRINK

Staying hydrated is vital for cancer patients. Dehydration can lead to abnormalities in the electrolytes in the patient's body, particularly if the patient has diarrhea. I encourage patients to drink water throughout the day.

If a patient has pain from sores in the mouth and finds it hard to swallow, inform the medical team right away. Some medicines can help with pain to improve swallowing. We want to make sure patients can continue to get liquids down.

If a patient is unable to swallow enough liquids, we sometimes provide fluids through a vein. This is known as receiving *IV fluids*. We give these fluids to help maintain a patient's blood pressure. This makes sure there's enough blood flow to vital organs, such as the brain.

HIGH-CALORIE SUPPLEMENTS

If a patient isn't eating enough solid or liquid foods, doctors often suggest adding a nutritional supplement to their diet. Boost and Ensure are common supplements, as they're high in calories.

Some patients lose weight even if they're taking most food by mouth. In that situation, adding in one or two of these supplemental drinks a day can help patients keep weight on.

During the hard parts of cancer treatment, many patients find it difficult to swallow any solid food. Doctors may suggest drinking three to six cans of these supplements to get enough calories.

It's important to determine how many supplements a day a patient needs to maintain weight. This depends on how much they're eating and drinking. As mentioned before, to maintain weight, a patient should try to take in 1,200 to 1,500 calories a day.

Many clinics can help patients get these supplements in bulk.

FEEDING TUBES

With different types of cancer treatment, sores can develop in the mouth and throat, making it painful to swallow. This can make eating hard and make keeping weight on a challenge. The medical team should decide whether a feeding tube is needed to help maintain nutrition. If a patient needs a feeding tube, doctors place it in an outpatient (go-home-the-same-day) procedure.

A *feeding tube* enters the stomach directly. The tube is sometimes called a G-tube, where *g* stands for "gastric." A patient can then put special food directly into the tube. Most patients tolerate a feeding tube well. Nurses and doctors can help a patient learn how to use it.

Once cancer treatment has started, getting a feeding tube placed can lead to an interruption in treatment, which isn't a good thing. Often, if a feeding tube is placed during treatment, it's because a patient is losing too much weight.

It's best to get a feeding tube in place before a significant amount of weight is lost! It's always easier to keep up weight during cancer treatment than to play catch up.

FIBER: FRIEND AND FOE

When a patient isn't undergoing cancer treatment, high-fiber foods are considered an important part of a healthy diet. Fiber is from plants that aren't easily broken down by enzymes (proteins) in the gut. These materials absorb water and other materials and help digestion by causing an increased bulk (volume) of stool. In fact, high-fiber diets—with oatmeal, vegetables, fruits, and the like—may lead to a lower risk of colon cancer.

During cancer treatment, some patients poorly tolerate high-fiber foods. They may have cramping and diarrhea, which may be due to increased motility (the bowel moving stool forward at a faster rate).

Some providers suggest starting out with a low-fiber diet during cancer treatment. Remember, there's no "right" answer regarding fiber during cancer treatment. Diets may change depending on the patient's specific situation.

SHOULD I AVOID SUGAR?

Many people are interested in the idea of limiting sugar during and after cancer treatment. Why? This stems from the Warburg effect (see chapter 2)—the observation that cancer cells pick up and use sugar at a faster rate than normal cells in the body. Cancer cells are dividing more often and need more energy to grow. Thus they need more sugar!

If cancer cells need more sugar, shouldn't you limit sugar in order to starve them? The short answer is no. There are a few reasons not to limit sugar during treatment. The first is that there's limited clinical evidence of any benefit.

The amount of sugar you take in doesn't have much effect on the amount of sugar in your blood. Hormones in the blood—insulin and glucagon—help keep steady levels of sugar in the bloodstream. These hormones make sure sugar levels don't get too high or too low. This is regardless of how much sugar you take in (unless you have a condition such as diabetes). The body does this because many organs, such as the brain, need a steady supply of sugar.

Limiting sugar may limit a patient's calorie intake. It's worth repeating: Patients do worse if they lose weight during cancer treatment. A cancer patient undergoing treatment needs to keep up their weight. I want to make sure a patient continues to get enough calories. The ideal is a balanced diet (the Mediterranean approach I mentioned earlier), but I wouldn't be upset if a patient got significant calories from sugar during treatment.

I will say that some research suggests that in treating cancer there *may* be a benefit to a ketogenic diet. A *ketogenic diet* is high in fat and includes some protein but little sugar. The benefit is unclear, and research is ongoing.

THE ROLE OF VITAMINS

Data is lacking on the role of vitamins during cancer treatment. I tell patients that once-daily multivitamins are likely fine during or after cancer treatment.

In theory, during cancer treatment, the antioxidant effect of multivitamins could work against radiation or chemotherapy. Remember, radiation makes oxidants, which damage the DNA of cancer cells. Vitamins are antioxidants and could work against these treatments. But this idea is theoretical, and little data exists. Many providers still support taking a daily multivitamin during cancer treatment.

What about separate supplements? Excessive doses of vitamin A (beta-carotene), selenium, and vitamin E are not recommended before, during, or after treatment. They do not protect against cancer and may even put patients at risk for certain cancers. Also, high-dose vitamin C may work against cancer treatments, such as radiation and chemotherapy! (See chapter 10 on complementary medicine for details.)

The takeaway? I don't recommend excessive high doses of any particular vitamins. A daily multivitamin is likely fine.

ALCOHOL: MAKING SIDE EFFECTS WORSE

Alcohol is bad for both organ and brain function.

There's evidence that one glass of red wine a day (as part of the Mediterranean diet) may be helpful for heart health. However, this benefit has become increasingly questioned. Excessive alcohol intake can put a patient at risk for a variety of cancers, such as liver and throat cancer. Because alcohol contributes to obesity, it may indirectly raise the risk of other cancers, such as breast or uterine cancer.

Drinking alcohol during cancer treatment is not recommended. Many treatments, like chemotherapy or radiation, make the tissues raw. Think of scraping your knee: How would you feel if you poured rubbing alcohol on a scraped knee? It hurts! Now imagine doing that inside your body when you combine alcohol and cancer treatment. Not a good idea.

If cutting down on alcohol is difficult for you or a patient, seek help through your emotional support team. There are medications and support groups to help patients quit drinking.

QUIT SMOKING—IT'S THE BEST THING YOU CAN DO!

There's so much data that smoking is bad for you that I can't overstate the risk. Smoking puts you at risk for cancer, heart disease, stroke, and other diseases.

Clinical data shows that patients who smoke during cancer treatment experience worse side effects than nonsmokers. Lung cancer patients who continue to smoke during chemotherapy and radiation have more problems with swallowing and coughing. In fact, if you have lung cancer and you keep on smoking through treatment, you're less likely to survive!

Quitting tobacco is one of the most powerful things you can do to improve your health. It can improve your chances of surviving cancer, make you less likely to get a second cancer, and help you live longer.

That doesn't mean quitting is easy. Even Sigmund Freud, the famous neurologist and psychologist, couldn't quit tobacco! But there is help. Reach out to your doctors to discuss options for quitting. There are tons of resources, such as nicotine gum, nicotine patches, medications, and support groups. I want to make special note of other types of tobacco: chew, vaping, and e-cigarettes. We know that chew leads to cancer of the mouth and jaw and is not a safe alternative. We will discuss vaping next.

VAPING: NOT A SAFE ALTERNATIVE

Vaping and e-cigarettes *are not* a safe alternative to cigarettes. Vaping is one of the most commonly used tobacco products among youth. This is because different flavors are available and it's advertised as a "healthier" alternative to cigarettes. Although long-term data is lacking, there are some chemicals in e-cigarettes and vaporizers that are cancer-causing. There is also a concern that younger people starting with vapes or e-cigarettes are more likely to start smoking regular cigarettes.

Some patients ask about vapes or e-cigarettes as a bridge to help stop smoking. If vaping or e-cigarettes can be used as a bridge to stop smoking altogether, I would recommend using them for the short term. However, they are not a long-term safe option.

1-2-3 EXERCISE

Exercise is critical before, during, and after a diagnosis of cancer. Exercise is part of maintaining a healthy body weight, which also affects a patient's risk of cancer. Proper exercise boosts the immune system, lowers the risk of heart attack, improves mood, and supports muscle mass. Regular exercise may allow some patients to bounce back faster after cancer treatment. Many medical organizations now recommend exercise as part of the cancer treatment! (https://www.cosa.org.au/media/332488/cosa-position-statement-v4-web-final.pdf).

Some data shows that even an eight-minute workout can decrease tension and anger. When you exercise, your body releases natural painkillers (endorphins) that help improve mood and increase happiness. By exercising, you also improve your sleep—something many cancer patients struggle with.

How much should you exercise as a cancer patient? I recommend about 20 to 30 minutes of aerobic exercise three to four times a week, as tolerated. This means a lot of things for different people. Exercise for some may be a walk around the block. For others, it may be biking a few miles.

The key is not—I repeat *not*—overdoing it. If a patient pushes too hard and too fast, it could make it hard to get through treatment. Patients need to listen to their bodies to find their limits.

Physical therapy (PT) and occupational therapy (OT) are services to help improve activity and mobility. They're terrific ways to support strength during and after cancer treatment. The use of PT and OT services can make a big difference in arm or leg function, especially if there's swelling. Every doctor loves a patient who is interested in maintaining activity through PT and OT!

Cancer treatment can be exhausting, making it hard to get enough exercise. You can read about dealing with fatigue in the next chapter.

GETTING ZZZ'S

Sleep is an often-overlooked aspect of cancer care. A good night's sleep can help relieve stress, tension, headaches, and other symptoms.

Sleep can be hard to come by, given everything patients are going through. The side effects of treatment, the stress of the diagnosis, and a host of other factors may all limit sleep.

There are medications to help with sleep. But before jumping to medications (which have side effects), I suggest following a few tips on sleep. First, try to get regular exercise. Second, do something you find relaxing, such as meditating or listening to music. You can also practice good sleep habits, such as these:

- Get in bed only if you intend to go to sleep. Don't hang out in bed.
- Make sure to turn off the lights and TV when you get into bed. Don't watch TV or use your tablet or smartphone in bed.
- Try to go to sleep at the same time each evening.

If a patient has a hard time getting to sleep, I have a few (nonscientific) recommendations: drinking decaffeinated tea with honey before bed works wonders. Some patients also benefit from soft music at bedtime.

If those don't work, melatonin helps some patients. Melatonin is a substance normally made by the body during sleep. It may be bought as a supplement over the counter, but patients should talk to their doctor before taking it.

CHOOSING TO MAKE LIFESTYLE CHANGES

Positive lifestyle changes help patients navigate cancer treatment and beyond. Many patients don't make these changes This leads to worse outcomes in the short and long term. This is the next common mistake patients make.

Mistake #9: Ignoring important lifestyle changes during cancer treatment that would improve outcomes and manage side effects of treatment

Of course, certain effects of cancer can make it difficult to make healthy choices. In the next section, we address some of these challenges head on: fatigue and cognitive difficulties.

DEALING WITH FATIGUE AND TROUBLE CONCENTRATING

A patient faces many challenges when dealing with a cancer diagnosis. As mentioned before, building a care team is critical, as it helps many patients deal with some of the side effects of cancer and its treatment.

Even though they have a team watching them through treatment, patients should understand some of the common effects of cancer. Some of these include fatigue and trouble concentrating. Understanding these effects will help patients deal with them and be their own advocates.

WHY AM I SO TIRED?

Fatigue is one of the most common complaints of patients with cancer. Surgery, chemotherapy, radiation, and immunotherapy all may cause fatigue. The cancer itself may also be a cause.

Why does it happen? No one is entirely sure. Treatment, emotional stress, the cancer, and a lack of proper nutrition are all likely contributing factors.

FINDING REVERSIBLE CAUSES OF FATIGUE

To treat fatigue, doctors first look for causes that are easier to fix. For example, we look for low blood counts. Emotional concerns and sleep problems also contribute to fatigue. Patients should work with friends, a counselor, or family members to discuss and work through emotional challenges (see chapter 4).

Exercise improves fatigue by reducing stress and improving sleep. Twenty to thirty minutes of aerobic exercise about three to four times per a week may improve mood, outlook, and fatigue. But a patient must be cautious to not overdo exercise, as this could backfire and make fatigue worse. As mentioned in the preceding sections, proper nutrition may help improve fatigue.

MANAGING FATIGUE SYMPTOMS

In terms of managing fatigue, follow the four Rs: rest, rejuvenate, remember, and reconsider:

- *Rest*: Make sure to get proper sleep each night. Try to find ways to decrease stress. This may include reading a book, setting up good sleep habits, or taking short naps throughout the day as needed. If you want to feel well rested, taking a few short naps is often better than one long nap.
- *Rejuvenate*: Find ways to restore your energy through music, time with loved ones, meditation, or other activities.
- *Remember*: Remember to pace yourself! A patient may become overly tired if they push too hard too fast.
- *Reconside*: If something isn't working, always consider other ways to improve fatigue. Don't get stuck doing one thing just because you've always done it that way. Keep trying new things until something improves your energy and mood. This may include planning out your day and trying new activities.

TROUBLE CONCENTRATING AND MEMORY PROBLEMS

Concentration problems and cognitive difficulties are common during and after cancer treatment. This can include problems with memory or mental cloudiness. Such problems may be associated with radiation to the brain (often whole-brain radiation) or chemotherapy ("chemo brain").

Other factors that affect memory and concentration include cancer itself, some antinausea medicines, age, steroids, trouble sleeping, depression, anxiety, hormonal changes, or infection. Realize that if you have trouble thinking, you are not "idiotic" or "crazy." These changes to the brain are real and can be hard for some patients to deal with. Still, most patients end up finding ways to cope and move forward.

RADIATION AS THE CULPRIT

Once cancer has spread to the brain, radiation often becomes a principal part of treatment. If radiation is given to the entire brain, patients may notice changes in short-term memory. This may be from radiation's effects on the brain itself or its effects on blood flow to parts of the brain. These changes take place months after radiation treatment. (If memory changes are occurring earlier, they may be due to the cancer or other changes in the brain.)

Most often, short-term memory is affected by radiation while long-term memory stays intact. Memory problems can be basic things like forgetting where your keys are. For some patients, the change is more significant: some forget what they did all day yesterday.

There are new radiation techniques to treat part of the brain while sparing the memory center (hippocampus). They're under study in clinical trials. Certain Alzheimer's medications (such as *memantine*) have also been shown to decrease the cognitive effects of whole-brain radiation.

Techniques and medications are always evolving, so talk to your doctor to discuss ways to decrease the effects of radiation on the normal brain.

CHEMOTHERAPY AS THE CULPRIT

Researchers haven't been able to consistently track the cognitive effects of chemotherapy on the brain. But this is probably due to a lack of standard ways of measuring these effects.

Chemotherapy may affect cognitive function by disrupting the *blood-brain barrier* (a wall around the brain that helps protect it). This is only one theory so far. The severity of the effect on cognition (thinking) may depend on other factors as well, such as depression and anxiety. Data is lacking at this time.

Patients may experience these effects in subtle or significant ways. Some patients have memory blocks, trouble concentrating, or the inability to juggle multiple tasks.

Because the effects of chemotherapy on the brain are poorly understood, there are limited treatments available. Helpful treatments include relaxation exercises, meditation, brain exercises (see the next section), and maybe some Alzheimer's medications.

WAYS TO MANAGE CLOUDY THINKING

A variety of techniques are used to help manage the way cancer and its treatments can cloud thinking. To support memory, don't overburden someone undergoing cancer treatment. Try to limit their mental workload. Ensure that the patient makes lists and that their days revolve around routines.

Family and friends or visiting nurses can help patients get things done around the house or help out with medications. The four Rs of fatigue may also help improve thinking (see the earlier section, "Managing Fatigue Symptoms").

Try to keep the mind engaged. The mind is like a muscle, in that if you don't use it, you lose it. Play board games, try puzzles, play Sudoku, or challenge a family member to a game of chess. It doesn't matter how you do it—just keep the brain engaged.

Working out the brain can be just as exhausting as working out a muscle. Patients need to get plenty of rest and eat brain food such as fruits and vegetables.

There's minimal clinical data on how to support the management of confusion and cloudy thinking for cancer patients. The approaches I describe come from individual experiences rather than research.

FERTILITY AND SEXUALITY

Many patients and families are understandably focused on survival and treatment after a diagnosis of cancer. But both fertility and sexuality are important parts of life. By thinking about these issues early on, a patient is better equipped to move forward with their partner after cancer.

FAMILY PLANNING AND CANCER TREATMENT

If you're interested in having a family after cancer treatment, discuss this with the doctors before the treatment is determined.

There's often significant fear and anxiety surrounding conception and family planning after a cancer diagnosis. This is because some chemotherapy, radiation, surgery, and immunotherapy treatments may harm eggs and sperm, leading to fertility issues.

Not all treatments cause fertility problems. Some cancer treatments may temporarily shut down the action of the ovaries, where eggs come from. These organs may regain function once the treatment is stopped. Other drugs shut down an ovary or testicle permanently.

Please know that many cancer centers have fertility experts that can help patients and partners with family planning.

FACTORS AFFECTING FERTILITY AND HORMONE LEVELS

Age at the time of treatment, dose of chemotherapy, and choice of chemotherapy regimens may all affect a patient's fertility. Certain drugs (for example, *cyclophosphamide*, *melphalan*, and *procarbazine*—see glossary) are more associated with infertility issues than others. Patients should discuss side effects of chemotherapy with their medical oncologist.

If radiation is part of the treatment plan, the dose to the ovary or testicle can affect its ability to produce hormones in the future. Radiation to female or male organs may impede a patient's ability to make hormones and/or carry a child.

There are surgical techniques to move ovaries out of the pelvis if radiation is being planned to this region. This may allow women to maintain function of the ovary. Young women (premenopausal) should discuss this option with their treatment team (for some cancers if the ovary is moved, there may be a higher risk of the cancer coming back; it depends on the type of cancer).

TECHNIQUES FOR FAMILY PLANNING

If a cancer treatment will likely influence fertility, patients and partners can take some steps to increase their chances of having a family later on.

For men, sperm may be frozen before treatment to save for later use; this is called *cryopreservation*. But note that cryopreservation may be costly and isn't often covered by insurance, and the donor has to be past puberty.

Some medications (leuprolide or *goserelin*) are thought to protect the ovaries from cancer treatment. They do this by shutting down the ovaries for a period of time. Why does this work? We know that chemotherapy or radiation works on rapidly dividing cells. If we temporarily shut down the ovaries, the cells are no longer rapidly dividing. These cells don't accumulate as much damage from treatment.

There are also early studies on egg freezing, but its long-term viability isn't well documented. This procedure is becoming more common, and techniques continue to improve.

If a female patient has a male partner or would like to use a sperm donor, freezing embryos is another option. This may allow a patient to pursue a family later on through in vitro fertilization (IVF).

The time dedicated to inducing ovulation (releasing an egg) and harvesting an egg must be weighed against the risk of the cancer progressing during that time. This process can take two to six weeks, depending on a woman's last period, which may be a long time in the context of a cancer. IVF or egg freezing may not be covered by certain insurances and can cost thousands of dollars. It is important to see what benefits you or your family have through the insurance company; your social worker may be able to help you do this.

CANCER CENTERS OFTEN HAVE EXPERTS ON SEXUALITY

Many cancer centers have experts who specialize in sexuality. Sexuality is a key aspect of patient care that often gets ignored. Supporting a healthy sex life (whatever that means for a particular person) will help them be happy and healthy moving forward.

SEX DURING CANCER TREATMENT

Sex may continue during many types of cancer treatment.

Many cancer patients experience a decreased sexual drive, fatigue, or other factors that affect desire for sexual activity. For both partners, understanding each other's point of view is important so that neither one feels lonely or physically isolated during the treatment.

Doctors suggest avoiding oral or anal sex during some chemotherapy treatments. This is due to the risk of infection. You can speak to your doctor about this.

Patients should also use contraception to prevent pregnancy during cancer treatment. Treatment with chemotherapy or radiation can have harmful effects on a growing fetus. This could include slow fetal growth, premature birth, or fetal defects or death.

SEX AFTER CANCER TREATMENT

After cancer treatment, regaining the desire for sexual activity may take some time—weeks to months. Side effects of cancer treatment may include erectile dysfunction, vaginal dryness, or other symptoms that make sex uncomfortable. Vaginal dilators, lubricants, and medications may help a patient manage these side effects of cancer treatment.

Discomfort with sex combined with a lower libido can lead partners to avoid sexual contact. I've found that the partner without cancer is often fearful of hurting their partner during sex. This leads to stress on a relationship and a feeling of rejection by both partners. Open communication is key. This allows partners to express their concerns about sex to make sure it's enjoyable and avoid feelings of rejection.

Many cancer centers have clinicians who specialize in sexual function. Spouses, partners, and patients need to advocate for their sexual health.

Returning to a healthy sex life is only one of the components of a healthy lifestyle after cancer. In the next chapter, we'll review tips for significant others after a cancer diagnosis.

Chapter Thirteen

Tips for Significant Others

A cancer diagnosis is difficult for everyone—the patient, partners, family members, and friends. For partners (a wife, husband, boyfriend, girlfriend), the period of their life during which their partner is diagnosed and treated for cancer may be the most challenging point of their relationship. Unfortunately, the rate of divorce or separation during this time is high. The stress of the cancer diagnosis and treatment can worsen existing underlying problems in a relationship. The key to getting through this stressful time with relationships in tact is open communication, understanding, love, and compassion for everyone.

THE BURDEN OF DECISION-MAKING

Watching a significant other go through a cancer diagnosis and treatment is very tough. Many partners feel overwhelmed. They often feel anxiety over how to help someone they deeply care for make sound medical decisions. Decisions neither person may fully understand. They're afraid of making the "wrong choice" for their loved one.

Someone dealing with cancer often feels "choice overload." Although their doctors and medical team should help guide patients in medical decisions with their preferences in mind; ultimately, many patients turn to their partners to make the decision for them or help them decide. There are specific ways significant others can help their loved ones navigate cancer diagnosis and treatment. Be supportive; you may know your partner the best out of anyone. Ask key questions to help your loved one reach a conclusion that is best for them and for the family:

1. What is most important to you and our family?
2. Do you understand the treatment options? (Write out the options for each treatment on paper.)
3. Now that we have a list of options, what is the best case and worst case scenario for each treatment? Does this help us decide?
4. How do these options fit into what is most important to you?
5. Do we need to call the doctors or nurses to clarify anything?

It is important that patients and their partners communicate openly about fears, anxieties, and goals with each other. Only by being open and honest about concerns and fears can these fears be addressed. Hiding fears may increase anxiety and add stress to the relationship. You can tackle this process together—by being open with one another.

YOU CANNOT POUR FROM AN EMPTY CUP: BURNOUT OF PARTNERS

As a patient goes through treatment, their partners are of the "front lines" dealing with the side effects. This includes managing nausea, poor appetite, fatigue, and the many other issues that arise. The partner is often left as the main advocate and caregiver for their significant other. They are often the one calling doctors or nurses to help make appointments or get medications. They often help their love one take medications. There is a constant stress on the partners of cancer patients to be available to aid and comfort their loved one. However, coping with all of this can put significant pressure on a relationship and on a person. The partner can quickly burn out.

There are key ways to help prevent the burnout of partners of cancer patients. *Ask for help early and often.* The more responsibility that constantly falls on the partner, the more stress this may create on relationships. Reach out to the medical and emotional support teams to see if they can find ways to help relieve the stress. This may include scheduling a visiting nurse to help with medications and symptoms management, obtaining a hospital bed at home, and referrals to physical and occupational therapy, among other types of aid.

Family also plays a key role in helping prevent burnout of a patient's significant other. Can a family member stay with the patient so the significant other—the primary caregiver—have an afternoon off? Time away for self-reflection and "me time" for a partner or caregiver is a key component to help prevent burnout and decrease stress. I encourage all partners to work with family members, religious organizations (church, synagogue, mosque, etc.), friends, and the medical and emotional support teams to find time for themselves. This includes taking the time to exercise and eat right. Caregivers and partners cannot take care of their loved ones going through cancer treatment if they are burned out.

In that same context, finding time to be "a couple" is key. If the patient and their partner have children at home, try to find a sitter (grandparents, aunts and uncles, etc.) so you can go out to dinner or a movie (or enjoy some other date night). Finding moments of normalcy in this tough time may make all the difference for the relationship. Of note, patients going through cancer treatment may not have the energy to go out to dinner and a movie (see the next section). But even just going for a walk and sitting by the lake may relieve stress. Quiet moments and time together "away from illness" to be with one another are most important.

ANGER: I'M SICK

Caregivers, family, and loved ones may notice that those with a cancer diagnosis—or any serious illness, for that matter—are angry at times. This is understandable. People wonder, *Why did this happen to me?* This anger may also be directed at love ones during this time. This is known as *displacement* (see the glossary). In this case, displacement is targeting some other person or situation with the anger caused by a cancer diagnosis. For example, the person with cancer may get "mad" that their partner burned dinner. Previously, they may never have gotten mad if this happened. It is important understand that the person with the cancer diagnosis is not really mad at an "overcooked dinner"; they're angry at the diagnosis and are transferring their emotions onto something else. As a supportive significant other, it is important that you recognize this. Do not take the displacement personally. Try to support your partner's emotions and work through what they're feeling. Help them recognize what is really bothering them. Please understand not every person will be ready to talk through their feelings or recognize the displacement right away. This may take time.

WHAT YOUR PARTNER NEEDS TO DO VERSUS WHAT THEY *CAN* DO

A cancer diagnosis is life-changing. Surgery may limit physical activity (running, biking, e.g.). Chemotherapy, immunotherapy, or radiation may cause fatigue. All of these treatments may affect a person's ability to do activities they love. This may lead to anger and frustration, which may be directed toward their partner (see the previous section on displacement). As mentioned in chapter 12, consider the four Rs: the patient should rest, rejuvenate, remember, and reconsider. And find activities that fit their *current* abilities. Even better if they are activities you can do together!

I see conflict arise when a partner wants to limit the activities of their significant other with a cancer diagnosis based on a doctor recommendation. The partner with cancer does not want to listen. They'll often say, "I feel fine. It's okay!" A person with a cancer diagnosis often wants to feel like a *regular person* and keep doing all their normal activities. The person with cancer may feel like they're being treated like a baby when they're told they cannot do certain activities. This frustration comes from wanting to get back to a normal life. This often leads to anger. As a partner to someone coping with cancer, open communication is key. Express fears or concerns to each other. For example, say something along the lines of "I am afraid of you getting hurt doing that." The person with cancer may say in reply, "But doing this is important to me. I need to find joy in something." These conversations are often complicated and emotional. I encourage you to bring in members of the emotional support or medical teams to better understand these issues.

A PRESCRIPTION FOR A DAY OFF FROM CANCER

There are so many doctors' appointments, infusions, scans, blood draws, and other aspects of a cancer diagnosis that can overwhelm patients and loved ones. The treatment can take a lot out of those affected by cancer. Every person is often looking for moments of normal—what it's like to live without cancer. A physician named Dr.

Toby Campbell pioneered a key concept in managing cancer care. He writes his patients a prescription for a "cancer-free" weekend or day—where it's not about coping with the cancer but about returning to a sense of normalcy. Not every doctor will write their patients this kind of a prescription, but you should feel free to write it for each other. Give yourselves periodic days off from cancer.

FINANCES: PLANNING TOGETHER

Fear of the future often delays important conversations surrounding money. You and your partner should take a close look at finances together (remember mistake #5). There are a few important questions to ask:

1. Does the family have enough in savings to have one income or no income for a few months? How much savings will we have left over after treatment?
2. Will we have difficulty making mortgage payments? Car payments?
3. Do we have disability insurance (private or through work)? Can we file a claim (depending on how long treatment will last)?
4. How will our finances look long-term (over the months and years after diagnosis)?
5. Health care is expensive. How do we protect our finances and our children's future?
6. Do we have life insurance? Do we need to obtain it?

This is a perfect time to engage with the emotional support team, such as a social worker, to ensure you and your family are obtaining all the benefits possible through the hospital and your current insurance. I would also encourage families to engage with an accountant to plan for your financial future.

CHILDREN: WILL THEY UNDERSTAND?
WHAT TO TELL THEM?

Discussing cancer with children may feel overwhelming. What a child will understand about a serious illness depends on their age. Many children do not understand death—for example, that it's permanent—

until ages five to seven. The age and maturity of children will determine the exact conversations you and your significant other can have with them about illness. I advocate honesty among the family. Remember that there are resources—like the emotional support team, comprised of social workers, counselors, support groups—to help guide how to approach these conversations. A variety of books have been published on sharing this information with children. Some books for children are also available. I encourage you to connect with your emotional support team to see what resources they recommend.

Chapter Fourteen

Survivorship

Congratulations! You, your family member, your friend, or your loved one made it through cancer treatment. This is a major accomplishment.

The journey does not end here.

Cancer survivorship comes with its own challenges. This includes dealing with the long-term physical and emotional side effects of cancer and its treatment. Lingering fear is a part of that challenge. Will the cancer come back?

The goals for cancer survivorship include the following:

- Watching for new cancers or a return of the treated cancer.
- Coordinating specialists and primary care doctors.
- Promoting helpful treatments that can reduce the long-term side effects of treatment.

There are entire books and courses devoted to care after cancer. We'll cover just the basics here.

STAYING CLOSE TO YOUR DOCTORS

Doctors offer some general guidelines for follow-up after cancer treatment. These vary widely, depending on the type of cancer and treatment.

Typically, follow-up is done every three to six months during the first two years after treatment. This follow-up often includes a physical, blood work, and scans.

After the first two years, follow-ups are spread apart to about every six to twelve months. After five years, a yearly check-in is common. But remember, the schedule will vary based on the stage and type of cancer.

DEALING WITH THE LONG-TERM EFFECTS OF CANCER TREATMENT

The side effects of cancer treatment can affect a patient's quality of life. In the long term, swelling of an arm or leg or trouble with swallowing is a common challenge. A patient can work with their primary care doctor and medical team to try to ease these side effects. Doctors often give referrals to physical therapy or occupational therapy, direct home exercises, or suggest other helpful treatments.

Some cancer treatments (such as chemotherapy and radiation) may place a patient at a higher risk for other health issues, such as a heart attack or stroke. By adopting healthy habits, such as quitting tobacco and following a diet and exercise plan, patients may lower the risk of these problems. See chapter 12 for more info on lifestyle changes.

ADOPTING A HEALTHY LIFESTYLE TO IMPROVE LIFE AND REDUCE CANCER RISK

Patients play an active role to reduce their risk of cancer. For example, a good diet and exercise plan can help cut the risk that certain cancers will come back or that a new cancer will develop.

The risk that cancer will come back gets smaller the further out from treatment a patient gets. At five years or more, the risk of a cancer coming back is small but still isn't zero. Many survivors don't think about or make the right lifestyle choices because they're so focused on the cancer coming back. Once patients are many years out from cancer treatment, they may die from non-cancer-related issues.

Remember, patients need to take care of all aspects of their health!

This is one of the biggest mistakes patients make:

Mistake #10: Focusing only on the cancer and forgetting about overall health and well-being after cancer

To help patients balance all these factors, many cancer centers have survivorship programs. These programs help patients make follow-up plans, coordinate care, and reduce their risks by providing proper medical follow-up and interventions.

If your cancer center doesn't have a survivorship program, you can find a lot of resources through the National Cancer Institute (see the resources at the end of this book). I've also provided resources through my website at stephenrosenbergmd.com.

Chapter Fifteen

Health Care Providers
Entering Oncology

This chapter is for the professional entering the field of oncology. However, reading this chapter may benefit anyone. In this text, I offer advice as you take on the care of people with cancer. Many of you are newcomers to the care of cancer patients. I hope you find my advice useful.

THANK YOU

I want to thank you. You have made a career choice to help so many people in need. Families, friends, and those affected by cancer will need your love, compassion, and expertise. I know you will do your very best for all of them. Thank you from the bottom of my heart for your efforts.

HOW DO YOU MAKE THEM FEEL?

As you care for patients and families, you will witness amazing things. You will see people become cancer-free you'd never thought possible. You will lose patients unexpectedly. There is joy and heartache in the care of people with cancer. Embrace the difference between what is in your control and what is outside of it. Our impact on patients, friends, and family is so much more than the cancer outcome. How did they *feel* coming to us for treatment? Did you brighten their day? Did you go that extra mile? Although we will not be able to cure everyone, we can impact how they feel during their time with us.

It is the little things of everyday life that add up in either positive or negative ways. Do the little things for them (like getting a cup of water or a coffee for a family member) that positively impact patients, friends, and loved ones around you. Imagine if it were you or a family member affected by cancer: how would you want to feel coming to an appointment?

BE PRESENT

Cancer clinics can be busy, hectic places. You can often feel like you're getting pulled in ten different directions at once. However, when you are with a patient, try to be "present" in the moment with them. Some providers get accustomed to being around sickness and forget to be in the moment with their patients.

My favorite quote on this subject comes from Dr. Paul Kalanithi (his book, *When Breath Becomes Air*, is highly recommended; see the resources section at the end of this book): "In the midst of this endless barrage of head injuries, I began to suspect that being so close to the fiery light of such moments only blinded me to their nature, like trying to learn astronomy by staring directly at the sun. I was not yet *with* patients in their pivotal moments, I was merely *at* those pivotal moments. I observed a lot of suffering; worse, I become inured to it."

To be with people at these moments, I have a few recommendations. Always try to sit down in a room; standing gives the impression that you're trying to leave the room quickly. You should try to make eye contact with everyone in the room (not stare at a computer screen). If you need to give difficult news, try to turn your pager off so you're not interrupted (this may not always be possible).

You need to try to respond to emotional reactions: Do people in the room look confused? Do they look sad? Anxious? If so, pause what you are saying and try to address what you see. Be sure to acknowledge and validate emotions and concerns. When I see that the people I'm talking to are overwhelmed with information, I'll often stop and say, "This is a lot of information coming at you at once. I realize this is difficult. What can I help clarify?"

Other simple acts may make a world of difference to the people receiving your care; offering a tissue to someone crying or, as I mentioned before, getting someone a cup of water or pushing someone in a wheelchair to get somewhere (even if that's not your job) may make someone's day a little better. As you build a relationship with the people you are treating, a simple hand on the shoulder (or other physical contact) can be reassuring. However, the art of physical contact takes time to develop.

THAT EMPTY-CUP ANALOGY

As I mentioned in other chapters, those affected by cancer need to ensure they take time for themselves; this includes you! Take time for self-reflection—writing, painting, going for a walk. I encourage you to stay active and fit—eat right and exercise. Enjoy recreational activities with family and friends. Sign up for an intramural league. Please stay active and involved with those who love and care about you. This will help keep you energized so you can take better care of people. Just like the caregivers of cancer patients, you cannot pour from an empty cup.

KEEP LEARNING

We have a duty to patients and those who trust us with their care that we keep learning. Cancer care continues to rapidly change. The treatment of lung cancer today is not what it was even five years ago. This is true across many cancers. As physicians, NPs, PAs, nurses, or anyone else involved in the care of patients, we need to continue to grow our knowledge. Keep learning, growing, stretching, and asking questions.

Knowledge is important for the care of our patients. However, I hope you will practice medicine with this piece of wisdom (often attributed to Theodore Roosevelt): No one cares how much you know until they know how much you care.

May your career be full of joy as you share this journey with loved ones, friends, family, and many others.

Chapter Sixteen

Closing Comments

I hope you found the information in this book useful. I tried to give you an overview of cancer so you could see the forest, not just the trees.

If you'd like to know more, I've included a list of resources at the end of the book. You can find resources on my website as well (stephenrosenbergmd.com). There's so much information available online and in books. Always try to gauge where you're getting your information. Remember the ten most common mistakes people make—they are summarized at the end of the book for you. For the four most common cancers—breast, prostate, colorectal, and lung—I've also included ten questions to consider at appointments. These questions may help you clarify confusing topics if you are dealing with one of these cancers.

I wish you, your family, or anyone you know who's been affected by cancer all the love and luck in the world! You're not alone on this journey. We're here with you.

Chapter Seventeen

Breast Cancer

Ten Questions to Ask

Throughout this book I've outlined the ten most common pitfalls people make when dealing with a cancer diagnosis. The questions below assume you've already addressed these critical mistakes—like building a treatment team and addressing goals of care. The questions below are specific to breast cancer and may help clarify treatments and decision-making. I outline definitions in the glossary for any scientific and medical terms.

1. What is the receptor status of my cancer? Estrogen receptor (ER)? Progesterone receptor (PR)? HER2? Are my receptors favorable or unfavorable?
2. Should I undergo genetic testing?
3. Do I need additional imaging? (CT scan? Bone scan? Breast MRI?)
4. Would I benefit from an Oncotype Dx score? If I need chemotherapy, what type will I receive? What are the main side effects?
5. Would I benefit from neoadjuvant chemotherapy?
6. Are there treatment options for keeping my breast (a.k.a. breast conservation)?

7. If I am interested in breast reconstruction, what options are available? Do other nearby cancer centers offer different types of reconstruction? When would the reconstruction happen?

8. If I need radiation, am I a candidate for hypofractionated (short-course) radiation? If not, why not?

9. How do you decrease the radiation dose to my heart during treatment? What technique are you using? (This issue is especially important for women with left-sided breast cancers.)

10. Will I need hormone (e.g., tamoxifen or anastrozole) or targeted therapy? If so, how long would treatment go on for? What are the side effects?

Chapter Eighteen

Prostate Cancer

Ten Questions to Ask

Throughout this book I've outlined the ten most common pitfalls people make when dealing with a cancer diagnosis. The questions below assume you've already addressed these critical mistakes—like building a treatment team and addressing goals of care. The following ten questions are specific to prostate cancer and may help clarify treatments and decision-making. I outline definitions in the glossary for any scientific and medical terms.

1. What is the Gleason score (or Grade Group) of my prostate cancer? How many biopsies were positive?
2. What is my PSA value?
3. Do I need additional imaging? (CT scan? Bone scan? Prostate MRI?)
4. How do you classify my prostate cancer by *risk group*—very low, low, favorable-intermediate, unfavorable-intermediate, or high-risk?
5. Is *active surveillance* an option? If not, why not?
6. Are both surgery and radiation options for treatment? If I have not met with a surgeon (urologist) or a radiation oncologist, can I meet with one to discuss the pros and cons of each treatment approach?

7. How do you approach surgery for the prostate? (Open? Minimally invasive? Robotic?)

8. If I need radiation, will it be external radiation or internal radiation (brachytherapy?). If I need external radiation, am I a candidate for hypofractionated (short-course) radiation? If not, why not?

9. For the proposed treatment, what are the long-term side effects for erectile dysfunction, bladder dysfunction (urination), and bowel dysfunction?

10. Will I need hormone therapy (e.g., leuprolide) or chemotherapy? If so, how long? What are the side effects? Should I undergo sperm banking?

Chapter Nineteen

Colorectal Cancer

Ten Questions to Ask

Throughout this book I've outlined the ten most common pitfalls people make when dealing with a cancer diagnosis. The questions below assume you've already addressed these critical mistakes—like building a treatment team and addressing goals of care. These questions are specific to colorectal cancer and may help clarify treatments and decision-making. I outline definitions in the glossary for any scientific and medical terms.

1. Do I need additional imaging? (CT scan? PET scan? Pelvic MRI?)
2. What are my tumor marker levels (*CEA*)?
3. Should I undergo genetic testing?
4. Would I benefit from chemotherapy or chemoradiation before surgery?
5. How many cycles of chemotherapy are you recommending? Would I benefit from immunotherapy? If not, why not?
6. A newer approach for colorectal cancer is chemotherapy and/or chemoradiation followed by surveillance (no surgery). Would I be eligible for this approach? Why or why not?
7. What type of surgery will I need? Will I need a colostomy bag? Would it be permanent or temporary? Do you have concerns

about your ability to remove all of the tumor (that is, concern for leaving behind cancer cells—a.k.a. a positive margin)?

8. Does my tumor show microsatellite instability or mismatch repair? What does that mean for my treatment? Does my tumor show mutations in KRAS? NRAS? BRAF? What is the tumor mutational burden? What does that mean for my treatment?

9. If my cancer has spread outside of the colon/rectum (*oligometastatic disease*), would I still benefit from aggressive treatment with radiation or surgery?

10. Would I benefit from fertility preservation before any intervention (like chemotherapy, surgery, or radiation)?

Chapter Twenty

Lung Cancer

Ten Questions to Ask

Throughout this book I've outlined the ten most common pitfalls people make when dealing with a cancer diagnosis. The questions below assume you've already addressed these critical mistakes—like building a treatment team and addressing goals of care. The questions below are specific to lung cancer and may help clarify treatments and decision making. I outline definitions in the glossary for any scientific and medical terms.

1. Do I need additional imaging? (CT scan? PET scan? Brain MRI?)
2. Do I have small cell lung cancer or non-small cell lung cancer? If non-small cell lung cancer, what subtype (e.g., adenocarcinoma, squamous cell carcinoma, etc.)?
3. Do I need to have my lymph nodes sampled? If so, how do you approach this?
4. Should I have surgery? What type of surgery?
5. Would I benefit from chemoradiation before surgery?
6. If I get surgery, will I need chemotherapy and radiation afterward based on imaging? Could I do radiation alone or *chemoradiation* alone?
7. Would I be eligible for stereotactic body radiation therapy (*SBRT*)?

8. What techniques do you use to spare the heart during radiation treatment? Do you use *IMRT*?
9. What is the PD-1/PDL-1 status of my tumor? Would I benefit from immunotherapy?
10. Does my tumor have mutations in *EGFR*? *ALK*? *ROS1*? *BRAF*? Would I be eligible for targeted therapy?

The Ten Common Mistakes
Patients Make

1. Not knowing the name and stage of their cancer (see pages 28, 31, and 39).
2. Not seeking emotional and religious support early (see page 34).
3. Being afraid to ask questions (see pages 41 and 77).

   Note: This includes asking for clarifications on treatment, plans, and prognosis. Not asking leads to a lack of understanding of the goals of treatment (cure, pain relief, etc.). There are no stupid questions!
4. Being afraid to ask for a second opinion (see page 42).
5. Not discussing finances, wills, health care proxies, and other end-of-life issues with family, doctors, and friends before or soon after a diagnosis, regardless of cancer stage or potential outcomes (see pages 43 and 115).
6. Not asking for a copy of their pathology report after surgery or scan results (see page 52).
7. Not having an up-to-date list of medications and supplements for the doctors (see page 59).
8. Waiting until very late into treatment or until the end of life to involve palliative care (pain management) or hospice care (end-of-life treatment) (see page 91).
9. Ignoring important lifestyle changes during cancer treatment that would improve outcomes and manage side effects of treatment (for example, stopping smoking) (see page 100).

10. Focusing only on the cancer and forgetting about overall health and well-being after cancer (survivorship—heart health, sexual health, etc.) (see page 116).

Resources

I have limited my choice of resources on purpose in this section. Patients or family members with the diagnosis of cancer are on information overload. There is an overwhelming amount of advice and information online and in books. I encourage you to go to stephenrosenbergmd.com for resources.

The following websites and books can give you tons of great information to better understand cancer and its treatment.

Paul Kalanithi, MD, *When Breath Becomes Air* (New York: Random House, 2012)

Siddhartha Mukherjee, MD, DPhil, *The Emperor of All Maladies* (New York: Scribner, 2010)

American Cancer Society, https://www.cancer.org

National Cancer Institute, http://cancer.gov

NCI Office of Cancer Complementary and Alternative Medicine, https://cam.cancer.gov/

NCI Survivorship, https://www.cancer.gov/about-cancer/coping/survivorship

NCCN Guidelines (free information with registration), https://www.nccn.org/professionals/physician_gls/default.aspx

US Preventive Services Task Force, https://www.uspreventiveservicestaskforce.org

UpToDate (doctors' website—subscription), https://www.uptodate.com/home

ClinicalTrials.gov (a data base of clinical studies being conducted around the world), https://clinicaltrials.gov

University of Chicago's Radiation Oncology Education Collaboration Study Group Patient Education page, https://voices.uchicago.edu/roecsg/patient-education/

Cook for Your Life (diet advice), https://www.cookforyourlife.org

Douglas Hanahan and Robert A. Weinberg, "Hallmarks of Cancer: The Next Generation," *Cell* 144, no. 5 (2011), https://www.cell.com/fulltext/S0092-8674(11)00127-9 (an influential paper on cancer biology that is a deep dive into understanding the basic biology of cancer; most appropriate for readers with a science background).

Glossary

- *abscopal effect* The shrinkage of a tumor in the body in response to a different tumor being targeted for treatment. For example, if you destroy a tumor with radiation in the lung, a completely different mass in the leg shrinks. This effect may be mediated by the immune system.
- *AC-T* A combination of chemotherapy drugs—Adriamycin (A; also known as doxorubicin), cyclophosphamide (C), and paclitaxel (T)—used in treating breast cancer.
- *active surveillance* Monitoring cancers with repeat biopsies and/or blood tests as opposed to treating the cancers with surgery or radiation. Active surveillance is appropriate for only certain cancers, such as very low-risk prostate cancer, that have only a small probability of spreading and causing issues during a patient's life. For patients with these very low-risk cancers, monitoring the cancer may be just as good as treating it.
- *activity (in PET scans)* How much radioactive sugar is taken up by the tumor cells during the administration of a PET scan. Where a lot of sugar is present, the image lights up. This may show the amount of tumor cells in a region.
- *acute side effects* The unwanted effects of cancer treatment that occur during or shortly after treatment is finished (within one to three months after treatment).

- *adjuvant therapy* A form of cancer treatment (chemotherapy, radiation, or immunotherapy) given after surgery to further decrease the risk that cancer will come back.
- *advanced directives* A document defining medical procedures and other interventions a person may or may not want when sick or at the end of their life. See also *living will*.
- *ALK (anaplastic lymphoma kinase)* A gene that encodes for a protein-promoting growth in cancer cells. ALK may be mutated in lung cancers to promote cancer cell growth. It may be targeted by various drugs (e.g., crizotinib).
- *alternative medicine* Medications or treatments used in place of traditional medical care. Many of these alternative treatments are unproven and have high out-of-pocket costs. In contrast, complementary medicine incorporates additional techniques with traditional care to manage treatment or side effects. See also *complementary medicine* and *integrative medicine*. It is important to note many textbooks mix up alternative and complementary medicine.
- *anastrozole (Arimidex)* A drug used to treat breast cancers that are *ER/PR-positive* (see glossary) by lowering the amount of estrogen in the body. Common side effects include hot flashes and joint pain.
- *antioxidant* A substance that works against oxidants, which occur in the body and cause damage to DNA. Examples of antioxidants include vitamin C, vitamin E, and selenium. *Anti* means "against." See also *vitamin C*.
- *APBI (accelerated partial breast irradiation)* A technique of radiation delivery for breast cancer, involving implanting needles, a balloon, or using external radiation for shorter time courses (one to two weeks) while only treating part of the breast. Traditional radiation for breast cancer takes place over three to six weeks and treats the entire breast. Many women find shorter courses of radiation more convenient. In general, outcomes with APBI are similar to older techniques. However, not all women are eligible for this type of treatment. Ask your radiation oncologist.
- *apoptosis* The self-destruction of a cell. When a normal cell has been damaged beyond repair, it self-destructs to prevent mutations that lead to cancer.
- *asbestos* A material that was once used in buildings and ships as a form of insulation. It is now found in older homes and shipping yards. Exposure to asbestos may increase a person's risk of lung cancer.

- *benign tumor* A growth or mass that does not spread or metastasize to other organs.
- *biopsy* A tissue sample obtained with a needle or scalpel so that it can be examined under a microscope, which allows doctors to figure out whether a mass is cancer or normal tissue.
- *blood-brain barrier* The wall between the brain and the rest of the body that helps keep toxins and other harmful things from the brain. Unfortunately, the blood-brain barrier also keeps many potentially helpful cancer-fighting drugs out of the brain.
- *blood counts* A slang term for analyzing a patient's blood. It measures the blood's ability to carry oxygen, fight infection, and clot correctly.
- *bone marrow* Tissue within the large bones of the body (femur, spine, and so on) that produces the cells in the bloodstream, including red blood cells, white blood cells, and platelets.
- *bone scan* A scan performed using a radioactive tracer. Too much or too little tracer in a certain part of the body may mean that region has cancer.
- *brachytherapy* A type of radiation treatment that allows for the insertion of radiation directly into a tumor. This type of therapy can be delivered in many different ways (for example, through radioactive seeds or needles).
- *BRAF* A gene that encodes for a protein that works inside the cancer cell to promote growth. This gene is often mutated in melanoma, lung, and colorectal cancers. This mutation may be targeted by a few different drugs (like vemurafenib, for example).
- *BRCA1 and BRCA2* Two genes involved in the repair of a cell's DNA. People with a mutation in the BRCA1 and BRCA2 genes may be at higher risk for breast, ovarian, pancreatic, and prostate cancers.
- *breast reconstruction* Rebuilding of the breast after breast surgery to treat cancer. There are many types of reconstruction options to remake the breast: breast implant (e.g., saline implants) or flap reconstruction (using a piece of tissue from another part of the body, often the abdomen). The options for reconstruction depend on the type of surgery a patient underwent and what their body shape is like. It is important to time reconstruction appropriately to other treatments such as chemotherapy or radiation.
- carcinogen: A drug or substance that may cause cancer after exposure. This may naturally occur or be man-made.

- *capecitabine* A common chemotherapy drug taken by mouth. The body converts capecitabine to 5FU (5-fluorouracil). A cancer cell takes up 5FU and tries to use it in part of a process to copy its DNA. 5FU resembles a molecule needed for the structure of DNA, but it's a fake, so it causes the cancer to halt its DNA copying process.
- *cancer* An uncontrolled growth of cells. In most ways, cancer cells mirror the functioning of normal cells. However, cancer cells focus on growing at the expense of all other functions.
- *CEA (carcinoembryonic antigen)* A tumor marker that may be elevated in the blood of people with different types of cancers. Looking at changes in CEA levels may help indicate response to cancer treatment. CEA levels are most commonly tracked in colorectal, pancreatic, and ovarian cancers.
- *cell cycle arrest* The growth and development of a cell can be broken into phases known as the cell cycle. If a cell senses damage, it will stop at a certain point in its cycle to repair the damage. This stopping is cell cycle arrest.
- *cell receptor* Every cell has a membrane that separates it from the outside environment. On the surface of the membrane are proteins that receive signals from and send signals to the environment. These proteins on the cell membrane are known as cell receptors.
- *chemoradiation* Chemotherapy administered at the same time as radiation to make each treatment more effective at destroying cancer cells. However, giving two cancer therapies together may also increase the toxicity of treatment. See the lawnmower analogy in chapter 7.
- *chemotherapy* A drug (or drugs) used to target the killing of cancer cells.
- *chemotherapy course* The number of cycles of chemotherapy administered over time to treat a cancer. See *cycle of chemotherapy* for more information.
- *chronic myelogenous leukemia (CML)* A liquid tumor of the blood. This cancer used to have a high mortality rate, but with the drug Gleevec used as a targeted therapy, today long-term survival rates surpass 90%.
- *cisplatin* A drug used to damage the DNA of cancer cells. It is often combined with radiation to destroy cancer (see the lawnmower analogy in chapter 7). Side effects of this chemotherapy often include kidney damage and hearing loss.

- *clinical stage* A patient's T (tumor), N (lymph nodes), and M (metastasis) classification as determined by doctors, based on information from a physical exam and scans. The TNM is used to put a patient into a final stage or group. The clinical stage is given before any surgical intervention to remove the cancer or lymph nodes. See also *pathological stage* and *TNM*.
- *colostomy bag* A small bag that exits the abdomen (belly) that collects stool (poop) after surgery to the gut or abdomen. It may be permanent or temporary, depending on the type of surgery.
- *complementary medicine* Treatments such as acupuncture, massage, music therapy, or Reiki that help manage side effects and other aspects of cancer care. Using complementary medicine is part of the integrative-medicine approach to cancer care. It is important to note many textbooks mix up alternative and complementary medicine. See *alternative medicine* for more information.
- *complete lymph node dissection* The removal of multiple lymph nodes that may contain cancer; often 10 to 30 or more lymph nodes are removed, but this varies by the type of cancer or the site. The goal is to remove all the lymph nodes containing cancer within a certain part of the body. See also *sentinel lymph node*.
- *crizotinib (Xalkori)* A targeted therapy drug that works on certain mutations present in cancers (ALK and ROS1; see glossary) and may be used to treat lung cancer, lymphoma, neuroblastoma, and other cancers. Although this therapy may be effective for quite some time, resistance to treatment often develops.
- *cryopreservation* The process of freezing cells to preserve them for future use. Most often semen, eggs, or embryos are frozen for later use in fertility treatments.
- *CT scan (CAT scan)* X-rays used to construct a three-dimensional image of the inside of the body. These scans are fast but don't provide the same level of detail as an MRI scan. See also *PET/CT scans*.
- *CT simulation* A CT scan given to cancer patients in order to plan radiation treatment. This allows doctors to target the tumor while minimizing radiation dose to normal tissues.
- *curative treatment* A treatment whose goal is to cure the disease—to eradicate the cancer from the patient.
- *Cyberknife* A specialized machine that delivers focused, high doses of radiation to specific areas to damage cancer cells through the use of X-rays, while sparing normal organs.

- *cyclophosphamide* A chemotherapy drug used to damage the DNA of cancer cells. It's also used to suppress the immune system in the treatment of other conditions. Common side effects to cyclophosphamide include low blood counts, nausea, and bladder irritation.
- *cycle of chemotherapy* The combination of days of active treatment (when a patient is receiving the chemotherapy via pill or IV) followed by a few days of rest in the administration of a course of chemotherapy.
- *displacement (as it relates to emotions)* The inappropriate transfer of emotions (such as anger) onto other people. A cancer diagnosis may cause a person to feel angry or upset. Open communication is key to helping the patient deal with the cancer diagnosis and avoid displacing their emotions onto others.
- *distant disease (spread)* The movement (metastasis) of cancer beyond its original site (where it originated), farther than nearby lymph nodes, to a different part of the body—for example, colon cancer spreading to the liver or lungs.
- *DNA (deoxyribonucleic acid)* The genetic material housed in the nucleus of a cell. The code or sequence helps define the function of genes and serves as the "brain" of the cell. DNA is the primary target of radiation and many chemotherapy agents.
- *dosimetrist* A member of the radiation treatment team with special training to help determine how to deliver appropriate doses of radiation to the tumor.
- *doxorubicin (Adriamycin)* A chemotherapy drug that interferes with the function of DNA. It's often part of treatment regimens for lymphomas or breast cancer. Important side effects of doxorubicin include a negative effect on heart function.
- *dronabinol* A drug derived from the active components of marijuana. It can be prescribed to treat nausea and vomiting in some cancer patients.
- *durvalumab (Imfinzi)* An immunotherapy drug (antibody) that targets *PDL-1* (see the glossary definition). This drug turns on the immune system to help target cancer. Durvalumab is often used to treat lung cancer after chemoradiation.
- *EGFR (epidermal growth factor receptor)* A receptor at the surface of a cancer cell that signals the cell to grow inappropriately. Many cancer cells have mutations (changes in DNA) in this receptor that turn on this signal to grow inappropriately (allowing the cancer cell to grow more often). EGFR is commonly mutated in lung and colon

cancers. Certain targeted therapies such as Osimertinib (see glossary) attack mutations in this receptor.

- *electron* A small, negatively charged particle. In the treatment of many skin cancers, radiation oncologists may use electron particles rather than X-rays. With their small size, electrons do not penetrate deep into the body. They can only be used to treat sites near the body's surface.
- *ENT (ear, nose, and throat)* See *otolaryngologist.*
- *emotional support team* A team of people (doctors, nurses, religious leaders, palliative care providers, social workers, family members, and friends) who help patients and family members deal with the diagnosis and treatment of cancer.
- *end-of-life decisions* Decisions on how to approach end-of-life issues. An example is the desire to use an artificial breathing machine at the end of life even if there's no hope of recovery. These wishes should be discussed with family, friends, and the emotional support team members. They should also be discussed with doctors and documented before a patient becomes very sick.
- *EPOCH* A chemotherapy combination of etoposide, prednisone, Oncovin (vincristine), and doxorubicin used to treat lymphomas and other cancers.
- *ER (estrogen receptor) and PR (progesterone receptor)* Estrogen and progesterone are female hormones normally available in the body. These hormones bind to the ER/PR receptors on breast cancer cells. Hormones binding to these receptors send a signal for a cancer cell to grow and divide. Many breast cancer treatments (*tamoxifen* or *anastrozole*) try to stop the hormone from binding to the receptor.
- *feeding tube* A tube placed into the stomach to allow food to be absorbed by the gut. In cancer care, feeding tubes are often placed surgically through the belly if a patient isn't keeping enough weight on.
- *fiber* A material that comes from plants and isn't easily broken down by the human gut. Fiber tends to absorb water or other materials that increase the volume of stool. High-fiber foods include oatmeal and certain fruits and vegetables. High-fiber diets are thought to lower the risk of colon cancer.
- *fraction (of radiation)* Radiation treatment is usually broken into multiple treatments. Each radiation treatment is called a fraction. Breaking up radiation treatment into fractions may allow for better recovery of normal tissues.

- *Gamma Knife* A specialized radiation machine used to treat focused regions of tumor within the brain. This machine can deliver high doses of radiation with precision. Like most radiation machines, it uses X-rays.
- *gene* A region of genetic material that contains instructions for creating RNA and then protein. The protein leads to an action around the cell. See also *DNA*, *protein*, and *RNA*.
- *general anesthesia* A patient is put completely to sleep; this requires the use of a breathing tube. General anesthesia is commonly used for cancer operations.
- *genetic testing* An analysis of a person's DNA to determine if their genes may elevate their risk of developing certain diseases, like cancer. Some people may be at higher risk for cancer because of a mutation in their DNA. If a patient has many family members with cancer, doctors may consider genetic testing.
- *Gleason score (Grade Group)* A form of tumor grading for prostate cancer. After a biopsy of the prostate, a doctor decides how abnormal the cells look and rates them on a scale of 1 to 5. The more abnormal the cells, the higher the number of the Gleason score. There are often 8 to 12 pieces of the prostate to look at under the microscope, and the doctor reports the two most common abnormal patterns. The two scores are reported with a plus sign, with the number of the most common pattern listed first, and the numbers are added together. For example, a patient's Gleason score may be 4 + 3 = 7, where 4 is the most common pattern. The higher the total score, the more abnormal the cells appear in the biopsy, and the more aggressive the tumor. Because the highest score for each is 5, the highest total Gleason score is 10. Most recently, the combination score is now given a Combined Grade Group of 1–5. For example, a Gleason score of 6 (3 + 3) is a Grade Group 1. The higher the Grade Group, the more aggressive the tumor.
- *Gleevec (Imatinib)* A targeted therapy used to treat CML (chronic myelogenous leukemia) and other cancers by targeting the Philadelphia chromosome translocation. The use of this drug turned CML from a lethal cancer to a chronic condition.
- *goal of care* Before a patient begins any cancer treatment, the goal of the treatment should be agreed upon: curative (curing cancer) or palliative (relieving pain and discomfort). This helps with treatment decisions. There's often some overlap between curative and palliative treatments.

- *goserelin (Zoladex)* A drug used to suppress the production of the sex hormones (for example, testosterone). Cancer cells use sex hormones to grow. If we decrease the amount of sex hormones available, cancer cells grow more slowly.
- *grade (of a tumor)* A measure of how abnormal cancer cells look under a microscope. The more abnormal they appear, the higher the grade. Higher-grade tumors tend to behave more aggressively. More aggressive tumors often grow faster and may spread more often to other organs.
- *gray* The measurement of the amount of energy given to a tumor as prescribed by a radiation oncologist. A gray is equal to one joule per kilogram.
- *health care proxy* A person designated by the patient to make health care decisions on their behalf if they become unable to make their own decisions. The health care proxy is often designated in a living will or advanced directive.
- *hepatitis B* and *hepatitis C* Infections caused by viruses that can damage the liver and put patients at higher risk for liver cancer.
- *HER2 (human epidermal growth factor receptor 2)* A *cell reeeptor* (see glossary) expressed on the surface of cancer cells that helps them grow. HER2 is commonly seen in breast and esophageal cancers. There are specific drugs that target this receptor to block it— limiting cancer cells' ability to grow (e.g., trastuzumab, a.k.a. Herceptin).
- *hospice care* End-of-life care (the last six months of life). The focus of this care is quality. Early involvement in hospice has been shown to improve patients' quality of life when dealing with cancer.
- *HPV (human papillomavirus)* A common virus that causes warts. Certain HPV strains (subtypes of the virus) put patients at risk for head and neck cancer, anal cancer, and cervical cancer. Vaccines are available to prevent these infections that may cause cancer!
- *hypofractionated radiation* A type of radiation treatment in which a little extra dose of radiation is given each day of treatment compared to historical radiation standards. By giving a little more radiation each day, doctors can shorten the total length or course of radiation treatment needed for patients (sometimes decreased by one to three weeks compared to old treatments). This type of radiation is becoming more standard for the treatment of breast and prostate cancers, and outcomes have generally been good.

- *immunotherapy* A new treatment for cancer, using drugs that leverage the body's own immune system to fight the cancer by releasing the brakes on the immune system. However, these medications may have some significant side effects, as the immune cells can attack both cancer and regular cells.
- *IMRT (intensity-modulated radiotherapy)* A modern radiation delivery system involving changes in the intensity and angles of radiation delivery in order to minimize damage to normal organs. Many different types of machines may deliver this type of radiation (which is still X-rays).
- *induction therapy* See *neoadjuvant therapy*.
- *integrative medicine* The incorporation of complementary treatments (Reiki, massage, yoga, and so on) into standard cancer therapies for the benefit of the patient and family. See also *complementary care*.
- *isoform (protein)* Proteins that originate from the same gene with minor variations (with possibly different functions) that develop during the movement of genetic information inside a cell (DNA to RNA to protein). Examples include KRAS and NRAS (for RAS definition, see glossary).
- *IV (intravenous)* Given through a vein.
- *IVF (intravenous fluids)* Fluids given through a vein.
- *ketogenic diet* A diet high in fat and includes some protein, often excluding sugar.
- *KRAS* See *RAS*.
- *laparoscopy* A surgery that uses a camera placed through a cut in the belly to look at the organs or to help see a tumor or mass.
- *late side effects (aka long-term side effects)* The side effects occurring more than six months after cancer treatment (surgery, chemotherapy, or radiation). Sometimes side effects improve over time, but they often persist long-term.
- *leuprolide (Lupron)* A medication used to treat prostate and breast cancer, that decreases the amount of sex hormones in the body. Cancer cells use sex hormones to grow. Common side effects of leuprolide include hot flashes and insomnia.
- *linear accelerator* The generic term for a machine used to deliver radiation to treat cancer. This is an umbrella term; there are many types of linear accelerators.
- *liquid tumor* A liquid cancer for which there are no visible masses throughout the body; the cancer cells live in the bloodstream.

- *living will* A legal document expressing a person's wishes regarding medical care. This includes directions on end-of-life care, desire for organ donation, and the designation of a health care proxy. A living will should be made before a person is very sick.
- *lumpectomy (segmentectomy)* This is a surgery to remove a breast cancer but leave the rest of the breast intact. This surgery only removes a part of the breast—allowing for breast conservation. This differs from a modified radical mastectomy that removes the entire breast (see glossary for *modified radical mastectomy*). Many patients will need radiation treatment after lumpectomy. Ask your radiation oncologist.
- *lymphedema* The swelling (edema) that occurs in the arms or legs from damage to the lymph nodes by cancer, surgery, chemotherapy, or radiation. See also *lymph node*.
- *lymph node* These are small structure that are found throughout the body and are home to the immune system. Your body has hundreds of lymph nodes. They become swollen and red with infections. Lymph nodes are a common area for cancer cells to spread to.
- *lymphoma* A cancer involving the lymph nodes.
- *mammogram* An X-ray picture of the breast at different angles to screen for breast cancer.
- *margin* See *surgical margin*.
- *medical physicist* A member of the radiation treatment team who uses their MS or PhD in physics to help develop and safely deliver the radiation treatment plan.
- *mediport* See *port*.
- *melatonin* A molecule naturally released in the body that helps regulate sleep. Melatonin is available over the counter as a sleep aid.
- *melphalan* A chemotherapy agent that causes damage to DNA. Common side effects include nausea and a drop in blood counts, which may increase the risk of infection or bleeding.
- *memantine* A drug used to help protect memory. It may be used for patients with Alzheimer's or may be used with radiation to the brain to help preserve memory.
- *mesothelioma* A form of lung cancer associated with past exposure to asbestos.
- *metastasis* The movement or spread of cancer from one part of the body to another.
- *microsatellite instability* This is a change (mutation) in cancer cells' DNA and is caused by the loss of normal function of a DNA repair

pathway in cancer cells (called *mismatch repair*). With an inability to use mismatch repair appropriately, damage in the DNA accumulates. More DNA damage (that goes unrepaired) leads to higher rates of mutation in these cancers. Microsatellite instability is often seen in colorectal and endometrial cancers. Some tumors with microsatellite instability may derive more benefit from immunotherapy drugs than do other cancers.

- *mismatch repair* See *microsatellite instability*.
- *modified radical mastectomy* A surgery to treat breast cancer that involves removal of all of the breast issue. However, this surgery has fewer side effects than the more aggressive *radical mastectomy* (which also involves removing underlying muscle) and has similar outcomes. Modified radical mastectomy is still more aggressive surgery than a partial removal of breast tissue known as a *lumpectomy* (aka, *segmentectomy*) that allows for breast conservation (see glossary).
- *MRI (magnetic resonance imaging) scan* A scan that uses magnets to look inside the human body. These scans, which use a narrow tube, tend to take longer to obtain than CT scans. MRI provides the best visualization of soft tissue compared to most other scans.
- *MRI-Guided Radiation* A new technology that combines an MRI with linear accelerators to improve soft tissue visualization while delivering radiation treatment.
- *mutation* A change in DNA. Random mutations that happen over time may transform a normal cell into a cancer cell. Mutations may be caused by environmental exposures (such as smoking) or infections (such as HPV or hepatitis).
- *NCI (The National Cancer Institute)* A branch of the National Institutes of Health (NIH) that helps fund cancer research across the United States.
- *neoadjuvant therapy* A form of cancer treatment (chemotherapy or radiation) that takes place before surgery. Also known as *induction therapy*.
- *nerve-sparing surgery* An operation with the goal of leaving the nerves controlling that part of the body intact.
- *nivolumab (Opdivo)* An immunotherapy drug (antibody) that targets *PD-1* (see glossary definition). This drug turns on the immune system to target cancer cells. It is often used to treat melanoma, lung cancer, and kidney cancers.

- *non-small cell lung cancer* A type of lung cancer that may or may not be related to smoking in certain patients. There are multiple subtypes of non-small cell lung cancer, including adenocarcinoma, squamous cell carcinoma, and others. Treatment is usually some combination of surgery, chemoradiation, and/or immunotherapy. *Targeted therapy* (see glossary) may be used in patients with certain mutations (such as EGFR, ALK, ROS1, or BRAF).
- *NRAS* See *RAS*.
- *nuclear-medicine test* A diagnostic test using a radioactive substance or material, called a *tracer*, that is placed in the body. If an area of the body takes up too much or too little tracer, it may imply there's a cancer or other problem. Common nuclear-medicine tests include bone scans and PET/CT scans.
- *nucleus* The control center or brain of the cell. This region holds the DNA that directs actions around the cell.
- *oligometastatic disease* The limited spread of disease from the primary site (where the cancer started) to other parts of the body. There is no universal definition for oligometastatic disease, but it is usually considered to be a distant cancer spread to one to five sites. Depending on the type of cancer, patients with oligometastatic disease may have a better prognosis compared to those with widespread cancer. Oligometastatic patients may benefit (though data is limited) from aggressive treatment to each site of cancer spread.
- *oncologist* A doctor who helps diagnose or treat cancer. There are many types of oncologists, such as medical oncologists, radiation oncologists, and surgical oncologists.
- *Oncotype Dx score* A score on a scale of 0 to 100 rating the aggressiveness of a breast cancer as determined by the genetic analysis of 21 genes. This test helps identify which patients with breast cancer may benefit from chemotherapy. An Oncotype Dx score of less than 26 typically indicates less of a benefit from chemotherapy. However, the score cut-offs do vary by age. Please speak with your medical oncologist.
- *Osimertinib (Tagrisso)* A drug used to target an EGFR mutation that allows cancer cells to grow inappropriately. This mutation is often found in lung cancer patients who were never smokers. However, cancer cells find a way around Osimertinib therapy over some period of time. See also *EGFR*.

- *otolaryngologist* Also known as an ear, nose, and throat (ENT) doctor, an otolaryngologist specializes in surgery and the treatment of diseases of the head and neck.
- *oxidant* A reactive molecule formed when X-rays enter tissues and remove an electron from water. The loss of an electron is called *oxidation.*
- *paclitaxel* A common chemotherapy drug used to treat cancers such as lung, breast, cervical, and pancreatic cancers. It works by preventing cells from dividing (doubling). Paclitaxel was first derived from the Pacific yew tree in the Pacific Northwest of the United States but now comes from cells grown in a petri dish. Side effects of the drug include lung inflammation, diarrhea, and hair loss.
- *palliative care* Specialized care that focuses on relieving pain and other symptoms of cancer or other diseases. Early involvement of palliative care in cancer treatment has been found to improve outcomes.
- *pathological stage* A patient's T (tumor), N (lymph nodes), and M (metastasis) classification upon the surgical removal and examination of a tumor and lymph nodes. The doctor then places the patient into a final group or stage. The pathological stage takes precedence over the clinical stage, which came before the surgery (note that for staging purposes, biopsies don't count as surgery). See also *clinical stage* and *TNM.*
- *pathologist* A doctor who examines tissue under a microscope to determine what it is.
- *PD-1 (programmed cell-death protein 1)* and *PDL-1 (programmed death ligand 1)* A receptor and binding partner expressed on immune cells and tumor cells. When PD-1 and PDL-1 bind, the cancer is able to "turn off" the immune system and hide in the body. New immunotherapy drugs block the binding of PD-1 and PDL1 between immune cells and tumor cells. This allows the immune system to "stay on" and hunt down cancer cells around the body. Many drugs work on blocking this interaction, including *durvalumab, nivolumab,* and *pembrolizumab* (see their entries in this glossary).
- *pembrolizumab (Keytruda)* An immunotherapy drug (antibody) that targets *PD-1* (see glossary definition). This drug turns on the immune system to target cancer cells. It is often used to treat melanoma, lung cancer, head and neck cancer, and certain lymphomas.

- *performance status* How an individual is functioning globally in day-to-day life. This includes paying bills, cooking, dressing oneself, and the like.
- *Philadelphia chromosome* A particular genetic translocation of chromosomes 9 and 22 creating a fusion gene—BCR-ABL1—seen in CML (see glossary). This genetic change helps cancer cells grow and is targeted by certain drugs such as Gleevec.
- *photon* A form of electromagnetic radiation. The energy of a photon depends directly on its frequency. In cancer treatment, we use high frequency photons (X-rays) to damage cancer cells. See also *X-ray*.
- *placebo* A pill or treatment that has no effect but is sometimes used when testing a new treatment or medication. The placebo gives researchers something to compare against to figure out whether effects of the tested treatment are helpful.
- *platelet* A part of blood made in the bone marrow that flows through the blood and allows the blood to clot.
- *PET (positron emission tomography) scan* and *CT (CAT) scan* Two imaging tests often administered together, in which the patient is given a radioactive sugar, which is taken up by cancer cells. This activity can be seen on a PET scan, but the image is grainy. A CT scan is obtained at the same time to pinpoint where the activity is found in the body (where the tumor cells are active). See *activity (in PET scans)*.
- *port* A disk (about the size of a quarter) placed underneath the skin. The disk is connected to a tube pointed toward the heart and may be accessed by physicians and nurses to administer drugs or draw blood. A port is also sometimes referred to as a *mediport* or a *port-a-cath*.
- *port-a-cath* See *port*.
- *power of attorney* A person with the legal authority to act on behalf of another person in legal or financial matters. See *health care proxy*.
- *procarbazine* A chemotherapy drug that damages DNA. It may be used to treat brain tumors or lymphoma. Side effects include a drop in blood counts and vomiting.
- *prognosis* The course a disease will take.
- *protein* The workers of the cell at the molecular level that use instructions handed down by the DNA. The flow of information inside the cell is from DNA to RNA to protein. See also *DNA* and *RNA*.

- *proton* A large, positively charged particle used as a form of radiation treatment. Radiation oncologists use protons at special centers, often with a focus on treating children. There are some theoretical benefits to treatment for adults, but most studies haven't shown a benefit compared to traditional photon (X-ray) radiation.
- *PSA (prostate-specific antigen)* A tumor marker found in the blood of prostate cancer patients. All men (if they have a prostate) have a normal level of PSA, whereas it is often elevated in men with prostate cancer. Most often, the higher the PSA number, the higher the risk group for prostate cancer.
- *psychiatrist* A physician (MDs or DOs) who goes on to specialized residency training focused on mental health issues and disorders. They can help prescribe medications and therapy to deal with a cancer diagnosis.
- *radiation therapy* The use of high-power X-rays (photons) to treat cancer.
- *radical mastectomy* A surgery that was historically used to treat breast cancer that involves the aggressive removal of tumors and tissues, including removing the breast, the underlying muscle, and most of the lymph nodes in the armpit. Although the surgery is disfiguring, it was the standard treatment for breast cancer up until the 1970s. Now studies have shown that less tissue can be taken out with the same outcomes and fewer side effects, using a *modified radical mastectomy* (see glossary).
- *RAS* A cell signaling protein that is often mutated inside cancer cells to help them grow. There exist different types of RAS proteins (e.g., NRAS and KRAS) that are activated in different cancers. The letter in front of RAS indicates a different *isoform* of the protein (see glossary). RAS is often mutated in colorectal and pancreatic cancers. Mutations in RAS may make certain cancers more resistant to therapy (such as EGFR inhibitors; see glossary). The RAS mutation allows the cells to "escape" from EGFR inhibitors.
- *R-CHOP* A common chemotherapy combo used to treat certain lymphomas, consisting of rituximab, cyclophosphamide, doxorubicin, vincristine, and prednisone.
- *recurrence* The return of a cancer or tumor. A *local* recurrence refers to the tumor coming back exactly where it once existed. A *distant* recurrence refers to the tumor coming back in a brand-new location, often far away from where it once was.

- *red blood cell* A cell made in the bone marrow. It travels through the blood, carrying oxygen to the body's tissues.

- *red-flag symptom* A symptom of particular note to doctors, as it may indicate a more serious problem than a common medical issue. Red-flag symptoms are not specific for one disease or problem; they simply tell doctors to take a closer look.

- *risk group (prostate cancer)* The classification of a prostate cancer's aggression as determined by PSA level, Gleason score (Combined Grade Group), number of biopsies involved, and any sign of distant disease (metastatic disease), which in turn helps us determine the right treatment strategy. The risk groups, as specified by NCCN guidelines, are very low risk, low risk, favorable-intermediate, unfavorable-intermediate, high risk, very high risk, and metastatic.

- *RNA (ribonucleic acid)* Transcribed DNA information in the cell nucleus. RNA then leaves the nucleus and passes its information on to proteins. Proteins are the molecules that perform the actions around a cell.

- *robotic surgery* A type of minimally invasive surgery in which robotic arms, controlled by the surgeon, help perform delicate tasks in an operation and allow for small incisions.

- *ROS1* A cell surface receptor that resembles ALK (see glossary) and promotes cancer cell growth. ROS1 is mutated in a minority of lung cancer patients. If someone has a mutation in ROS1, they may benefit from crizotinib therapy (see glossary).

- *SBRT (stereotactic body radiation therapy; a.k.a. SABR)* A form of targeted therapy delivering high doses of radiation (X-rays) to a very small area, with high precision. This form of radiation therapy is highly complex and can have millimeter accuracy. It is commonly used in the treatment of lung cancer and many other cancers. When SBRT is performed to the spine or brain it is called *stereotactic radiosurgery* (see glossary) but it is the same technique.

- *secondary cancer* A new cancer caused by radiation treatment (X-rays) or chemotherapy. When radiation is used to treat cancer, normal cells get a dose of radiation too. Normal cells usually repair radiation damage, but sometimes the radiation causes a mutation that isn't repaired. This mutation can lead to a new cancer. Some chemotherapy agents also cause damage to normal cells that is not repaired appropriately, causing a cancer. The risk of secondary cancer from chemotherapy and radiation is low, and it most often occurs years after cancer treatment.

- *seed and soil hypothesis* The assumption that certain cancer cells spread to certain parts of the body in particular patterns and that certain environments help different types of cancer cells grow better in these places (see chapter 1).
- *sentinel lymph node* This is the first set of lymph nodes to which cancer cells move. Sentinel lymph nodes are identified in surgery by injecting a radioactive dye into the tumor. The dye spreads to the lymph nodes, allowing doctors to then identify the radioactive tracer in the operating room to confirm which lymph nodes are the first stop.
- *seroma* A pocket of fluid that develops in a cavity in the body after surgery. To prevent the development of a seroma, drains are often placed into a body cavity after surgery to help remove collecting fluid.
- *small-cell lung cancer* A type of lung cancer most often associated with smoking. This is an aggressive lung cancer that tends to spread to the brain. Treatment is usually a combination of chemotherapy and radiation (surgery is rare).
- *solid tumor* A cancer that grows from any solid organ or structure in the body. Common solid tumors include breast, prostate, lung, and colon cancers.
- *stage* See *clinical stage* and *pathological stage*.
- *stereotactic radiosurgery (SRS)* A form of targeted radiation therapy delivering high doses of radiation (X-rays) to the tumors in the brain or spine. It is very similar to *SBRT* (see glossary), except that SRS is particular to the central nervous system (brain or spine).
- *surgical margin* A healthy rim of normal-appearing tissue around the tumor that surgeons remove to try to ensure that all the spread-out tentacles of tumor cells are removed. When pathologists examine a healthy rim of tissue, they look for tumor cells. If they don't see any tumor cells, the margin is negative. If there are tumor cells within this region, the margin is positive. A positive margin often means the cancer has a higher likelihood of coming back, but this is not always the case.
- *tamoxifen (Nolvadex)* A common drug used to treat breast cancer by blocking the effects of female hormones on cancer cells. Common side effects of tamoxifen include hot flashes and fatigue.
- *targeted therapy* The use of drugs designed to target the specific mutations (changes in DNA) that cancer cells use to grow to their advantage. Targeted therapies often work for quite some time, but

many cancer cells eventually become resistant. As a cancer cell becomes resistant, we may change to a different type of targeted therapy. An example would be the use of vemurafenib to target a mutation in melanoma called BRAF.

- *telomerase* A protein that protects the ends of DNA (*telomeres*) during replication. Cancer cells produce more than the normal amount of telomerase to protect their DNA, allowing them to grow and divide more effectively.
- *telomere* The protective ends of DNA that help prevent damage to essential parts of the DNA to grow. In normal cells, these protective ends get shorter with age (after each cell division). As a normal cell's telomeres get too short to protect essential DNA, the cell can't divide anymore and so it dies.
- *TMB (tumor mutational burden)* The measurement of the number different genetic mutations in a tumor. TMB is used as a biomarker for potential response to immunotherapy.
- *TNM (T-tumor), N-lymph nodes, M-metastasis) staging system* A method of cancer classification, where T depends on the size of the tumor or how far it invades, N depends on the number of lymph nodes involved and where they're found, and M is determined by whether a cancer has spread from one part of the body to another. See also *clinical stage* and *pathological stage*.
- *TomoTherapy* A specialized machine that delivers radiation in slices or pieces (*tomo* meaning "slice"). This allows doctors to shape the radiation to the tumor and spare other nearby normal organs. Like other linear accelerators, this machine uses X-rays to damage cancer cells.
- *translocation* Genetic changes that move different parts of the DNA (genome) near each other that are normally far apart. Translocation allows cancer cells to express parts of the genome inappropriately to help them grow or avoid cell death. These translocations may be targeted by some therapies (e.g., Gleevec targets the Philadelphia chromosome translocation; see glossary entries on Gleevec and the Philadelphia chromosome).
- *treatment binder* A three-ring binder or folder used to organize important medical information. Common sections to categorize the information include Medication List, Medical Appointments, Diagnosis, Pathological Reports, Scan Reports, Side Effects, and Other. Using a treatment binder can help patients and families feel organized.

- *treatment team* A group of expert clinicians working to help a patient decide on cancer treatment. The treatment team may consist of medical oncologists, radiation oncologists, and surgeons.
- *tumor* An abnormal growth of cells in the body that forms a mass.
- *tumor board* A meeting of doctors of various specialties (medical oncology, radiation oncology, surgical oncology, and so on) who review medical cases to come up with a consensus on how to treat a patient.
- *tumor marker* A protein that leaks out into the blood from tumors, which may be used to monitor reponse to treatment.
- *tumor suppressor* A gene that signals cells to stop growing. Just like the name implies, it suppresses or stops tumors from forming. The most well-known tumor suppressor, *p53*, is called the "guardian of the genome."
- *unresectable* The condition of being unremovable. Based on the location of cancer in the body, it may be impossible to remove the cancer because of damange to nearby critical organs. A cancer that cannot be removed by surgery is unresectable. Sometimes doctors give chemotherapy or radiation to shrink the mass (*neoadjuvant therapy*—see glossary) to help make it resectable (able to be cut out or removed).
- *urologist* A doctor specializing in the treatment of diseases of the prostate, bladder, or kidneys. Urologists often perform surgeries for prostate cancer.
- *vaginal dilator* An object inserted into the vagina to expand the vaginal tissues. A vaginal dilator helps prevent narrowing of the vaginal canal and is commonly prescribed for women who have had radiation to the pelvis. It helps maintain sexuality and allows for future cancer screening.
- *vemurafenib (Zelboraf)* A form of targeted therapy aimed at specific changes in cancer cells (BRAF) for patients with melanoma, colorectal, and lung cancers.
- *vitamin C* An antioxidant vitamin often used as an alternative therapy cancer treatment. There's no evidence that vitamin C should be used in place of standard cancer therapies.
- *VMAT (volumetric modulated arc therapy)* An advanced form of radiation delivery using a linear accelerator machine. VMAT has the advantage of shorter treatment times. Many different types of radiation machines can deliver VMAT, which still uses traditional X-rays (photons) to treat cancer.

- *Warburg effect* A cancer cell is inefficient in its use of sugar to grow. Therefore, it requires more sugar than the average normal cell. The need for excess sugar for a cancer cell to function is known as the Warburg effect. If you want to read a scientific discussion on the Warburg effect, you can find it here: https://www.ncbi.nlm.nih.gov/pmc/articles/PMC4783224/.

- *white blood cell* A cell made in the bone marrow. It travels through the bloodstream and is important to fight infection.

- *X-ray* A form of electromagnetic radiation invisible to the human eye. Special high-energy X-rays are generated by radiation machines (linear accelerators) to treat cancer. Low-energy X-rays are used to look inside the human body (CT scan).

Index

161

About the Author

Stephen Rosenberg, MD, is a radiation oncologist, researcher, and writer. In medical school he was named a Howard Hughes Medical Institute Research Fellow. He was also named Suzanne Munson Intern of the Year at Memorial Sloan Kettering Cancer Center and at the University of Wisconsin served as Chief Resident in Radiation Oncology. Today he is Assistant Professor and Director of the MRI Guided Radiation Therapy at the H. Lee Moffitt Cancer Center and Research Institute in Tampa, Florida, where he lives with his wife, son, daughter, and two dogs. He is an avid coffee drinker, art lover, fisherman, and traveler. You can connect with him at stephenrosenbergmd.com.

9 781538 134221